THE FIVE SECRETS FOR HEALING YOURSELF AND OTHERS

ഇഇൽ

Dr. Robin L. Futoran

Canoe Tree Press

Published 2019 in the United States of America
ISBN 978-1-7338050-0-1

For permission requests please contact:

Canoe Tree Press
4697 Main Street
Manchester, VT 05255

www.CanoeTreePress.com

For author contact:
http://drrobinlfutoran.com

For my Father, a Bright Spirit and Guiding Light of Love and Family.
As in Life and now Beyond,
A model for Living Life Fully in the Greatest Adventure, Health and Joy.

Table of Contents

CHAPTER SEVEN
A New Paradigm In Healing 203

Foreword

D r. Robin Futoran knows "FIVE SECRETS FOR HEALING YOURSELF AND OTHERS" and he's willing to share them with us. In the Introduction he sheds light on our current western medical system highlighting the restrictions, red tape, greed, unnecessary procedures and biased research that flood our market and taints our minds. Dr. Futoran states, "Rather than being a system of promoting health and caring in the best interest of the patient," modern medicine operates as an authoritarian business in search of mega profits at any consequence. He details diseases that are on the rise and practices that are malevolent enough to cause the reader to sit up and take notice of his poignant warnings. The good news is he points the way towards overcoming this medical monster machine shedding the cloak of the victim by becoming our own advocates.

He further encourages our innate ability to heal and shows us how we can promote our individual healing processes. For a start, he challenges us to shake our fixed notions of illness and embrace the greater possibilities for quantum level healing. Then he lays out the Five Secrets for Healing like a banquet of insider knowledge that includes the power for us to heal anything from a cut on a finger to cancer.

Delivering complex concepts in an easy to understand language, Dr. Futoran unites five familiar terms with a new, fresh perspective that when aligned as *"The Five Secrets for Healing Yourself and Others,"* are valuable to consider. Pertaining to medicine and illness, he questions: Is your knowledge accurate and true? Is your understanding limited by past experiences or outmoded concepts? Do you know that every thought or belief we have in our minds alters our bio-chemistry? Is faith only connected to religion for you, or can it be something more? He describes his version of *outcome* as a recipe for non-attachment to a preconceived result. Do those fit your beliefs, or might you have something to reconsider and expand in your thought patterns? He paints the way forward for each step towards the alchemy and synergy of healing.

Dr. Futoran's book courageously de-structures the mind and dissects how beliefs are created, especially around illness and health. He supplies us with the blueprints for constructing new ideas that are based on what we want to achieve in our lives and for healing. Cleverly, he illustrates his point by using novelist Leo Tolstoy and his story of the Three Hermits to make his case. Beyond this elegant use of rich Russian literature and not at the exclusion of other great thinkers, Dr. Futoran weaves quotes from excellent minds, past and present, deftly into his tome. Each quotation makes a prominent point that solidifies his theories.

Well written, the book flows from topic to topic fluidly with insights and Ah-ha moments on every page. It carries the reader along at a friendly pace and an even keel. His honesty is refreshing and in his own words, he lays out his primary intention for the book as, "Through alignment of the five essential components for healing, bringing yourself or recipient to a place of knowing without a doubt, within every cell of your body and within the energetic nature of energy who you are, that you can and will heal." The book is all about us, for us and to us with love, from Dr. Futoran.

Dr. Futoran is a seasoned medical professional with over 30 years of clinical experience in his own clinical practice. He writes from a place of educated knowledge and skill. There may be many books on the shelves that speak of alternative, holistic, healing, but his book stands apart because it is written with authentic care and concern for the reader. Dr. Futoran wants nothing more than for each of us to put the gifts of his vast knowledge into practice and save ourselves. From what? Well, you can fill in that blank after you read the book. You may need several sheets of paper for notes. I heartily recommend this book to anyone who wants to be healthy and live life in personal power. This book is more than worth your time; it could easily be worth your life.

Kac Young PhD, ND, DCH, CRMT

Preface

For most people, seeking medical care can be a highly frustrating and often ungratifying chore, leading them to ask, "why am I not responding to appropriately prescribed treatments when others with the same condition are cured?" What might appear as the proper path to healing may instead evolve into a maze of unending diagnostic testing and experiments of medications, surgeries and alternative therapies, sometimes helping and other times creating new medical issues. The time has come to revolutionize and expand the way you think and participate in your health and healing. You have here an opportunity to increase your innate ability in healing yourself and others.

By the time you finish reading this book, your genetic coding will have been permanently altered. You read correctly, the DNA in your chromosomes will have been permanently reformatted with more expansive, positive perceptions, activated mechanisms and new understandings for the way illness takes place and how healing occurs. Consciously, anatomically and physiologically you will have the opportunity to be revitalized in health and the way you heal from illness. *The Five Secrets for Healing Yourself and Others*, will be a guide to raising your *healing consciousness*, allowing not only greater understanding, but increasing possibilities regarding the way you think and behave around illness and health. Through practical exercise and practices, you will have the opportunity for releasing and reformatting many of the limitations and obstacles you may be carrying that diminish or prevent healing. By the end of the book, you will not only have gained tools to more easily heal yourself and others, but have practices that can bring greater health, longevity, fitness and life joy.

Thirty years before I could even say the word *healing* out loud, I was practicing at the most conservative end of my field as a chiropractic orthopedist. A chiropractic orthopedist is a chiropractor who, after the standard chiropractic studies, continues for another three years of post-graduate orthopedic training in non-surgical orthopedics and passes an additional set of grueling board examinations, then making commitments to a refined set of advanced codes and practices for patient care. I served on the board of an international chiropractic orthopedic organization in every chair, including as president and was ultimately appointed the organization's youngest advisor. I lectured at universities, conferences and to organizations across the country and internationally. As part of a small group of practitioners, I participated in the development of ultrasound imaging for neuromusculoskeletal applications, acquiring the first FDA approval on a portable ultrasound device for that specific use. My curriculum vitae is more than nineteen pages long and my practice was built on relationships with the best medical specialist in Los Angeles, California. This was accomplished when I first started practicing, by searching out the best specialists in each field of medicine. I made lunch appointments with them, building a relationship and making it clear that if their patients were not surgical candidates, meaning they were not in need of spine surgeries due to herniated discs, spinal stenosis (a narrowing of the spinal canal), repairs of ligaments in the knees, shoulders or wrists, that I had the knowledge and skills to conservatively bring them back to a healed and pain free state.

I share this part of my resume not to impress you but rather to describe my longtime, conservative clinical practice procedure and approach. Throughout most of my first thirty years in practice, I would never have mentioned words like *healing* or *energy* to patients and colleagues for fear they might think I had gone off the deep-end from my conservative clinical approach to treating patients, and rather veered off into a *metaphysical* woo-woo type of practice. But, at the same time, I had a secret! You see, under the veil of my clinical chiropractic orthopedics practice, I was in fact, additionally and secretly, *healing* patients! Oh my! In referring to healing, I am talking about practices and methods of restoring health to tissues and the body that are typically not accepted by the domain of medicine and healthcare. In other words, they are metaphysical systems of practice, representing approaches beyond the current ability of science to observe or prove them true through the present capabilities and limitations of testing equipment. This secret healing part of my clinical practice was taking place instinctively and spontaneously, based on teachings and experiences earlier in my life. I will better explain this here.

My interest in healing and healthcare began many years prior to studying medicine and chiropractic. In my youth, unbeknownst to my family, I was secretly attending classes on healing, reading auras and past life regression. All great metaphysical fun and valuable on so many levels for reasons I didn't understand at the time, especially considering in those days it was all practically considered witchcraft. As I saw no future in these somewhat forbidden magical arts of the day, I closed all the books, stopped attending the metaphysical courses, turning my focus back to school and the accepted sciences of illness and health. Having this early underlying knowledge based in metaphysical studies, lead me throughout my training, to always correlate the science of illness and patient care, to the unseen science and forces of energy. What I want you to understand here is that with all my training and credentialing in conservative methods of healthcare, I was also quietly utilizing metaphysical healing practices then based on science. Fortunately, since that time, many aspects of what I had practicing in healing methods have now been scientifically proven. This melding of knowledge and education in the physical sciences along with the knowledge, understanding and experience in metaphysical science is what generated the creation and production of this book.

Introduction

This is no ordinary time in addressing issues around illness and health. There is significant discord and corruption within medical system, including bias in research, restrictions and red-tape by insurance companies, greed in the pharmaceuticals industry and insurance companies, even unethical practices by some physicians and healthcare services generally. I cringe thinking of the frequent pharmaceutical television and radio advertisements marketing critical life-saving and at the same time, health threatening drugs, with potentially serious side effects, as if selling trivial hamburgers from a fast food chain. Too often the healthcare *business*, unfortunately, to flourish with mega-profits, often acts from the perspective of powerful authoritarians with unfairly principled practices in the development and marketing of drugs, rather than being a system of promoting health and caring in the best interest of the patient. And while great advances continue to be forged in medical sciences and some people are living longer, they are not living healthier, nor are they happier. Take cancer treatment for instance, while mortality outcomes in some cases have improved and only to a minor degree over the last fifty years, these patients who are living longer are most often sicker, having more disease and undergo unending treatment and care. Considering the United States is a world leader in medical innovation, it is not the healthiest or the happiest when compared to other countries. The U.S. is even far from the top ten. Depending on the study, compared to 188 other countries, the U.S. ranks between the 28th and 34th healthiest country, while being only 31st in life expectancy. On the happiness scale, the U.S. again fails to be in the top ten, sitting in a about 18th place. And in ranking the best medical care systems according to the World Health Organization (WHO), the United States rests at 37th.

Even with our great advances in medicine, we are witnessing an evolution of new diseases. At the same time, we see so many conditions that were once considered rare, becoming commonplace. In 2007, the WHO reported that infectious diseases were emerging at a rate never seen before. Since the 1970s, more than 40 infectious disease that were previously unknown or undetected have been discovered including Hantavirus (1993), Ebola (2014), Avian flu (1997), West Nile Virus in the U.S. (1999), HIV (1983), MERS (2012), SARS (2002), Swine flu (2009), Mad Cow Disease, and most recently, Zika virus.

In the same fashion, infectious diseases are mutating and becoming resistant to antibiotics and treatments that were once effective. New strains of the Influenza virus and Cholera have presented challenges to medicine. Tuberculosis, dengue fever, Zika, Influenza, Chikungunya disease, MERS and SARS are all on the rise. According to the Center for Disease Control (CDC) in a 2007 report, tick borne illness has been increasing over the last thirteen years at an alarming rate and expanding to locations that had never seen these diseases. In a recent report, cases of Hepatitis C had tripled, with hospitalization increasing by fifty percent, along with a marked increase in mortality. Tuberculosis, Hepatitis B and Shingles are recently on the rise.

Realizing the difficulties in meeting the challenges of new and resurgent disease, we are inundated through the media and Internet with volumes of misinformation overflowing at our finger tips on disease and health. People are visiting five different doctors who might offer five different opinions. When facing a health crisis, especially from a place of fear and worry, it is easy to venture down erroneous paths that lead to misdiagnosis and maltreatment, veering away from the best possible therapies and diverting from an ideal course of healing. At minimum, utilizing the healthcare system can be all too circuitous and frustrating.

But think about this, in the face of all these challenges in medicine, with the healthcare system often in turmoil, there are people getting better. Some are responding to standard medical care, others healing through alternative therapies and some improving with no treatment at all. It is conceivable as it takes place every day, that you or someone you know, might accidentally and even spontaneously heal from pretty much any type of disease. That is the subject of this book. Our innate ability to heal and how we can be an active participant enhancing and promoting the healing process.

By the end of this book, not only will you have reformatted your healing consciousness to more expansive possibilities in healing yourself and others, but there will be that permanent alteration in your DNA. Your mind and body will have altered its understanding of illness and how you "believe" healing takes place. This process unfolds through a physiological pathway is known as *Placebome Effect*, which you will learn more about shortly. My intention is that your ability to heal yourself and others will be greatly enhanced in ways you have never imagined. Whether you are aware of it or not, consciously or unconsciously, you have been healing yourself and other people for your entire life. We all have the capability for healing ourselves and it takes place more often accidentally through the process of whatever our life work or passion may be. You might be a doctor, an alternative healthcare practitioner, a healer, a parent, a business owner, salesperson, teacher, a police officer, singer, dancer, in the military, in food service, it matters not. Our ability to heal ourselves and others flows through the service and intention of our work and passions. As you will see, we all play a vital role in healing ourselves and others through the *energy of our thoughts*, feelings and emotions. Throughout these pages your healing capabilities will be expanding, growing and bringing you greater joy and pleasure in life.

Be aware, that everything *you think you already know* about illness and health is rooted in old, fixed ideas and information your learned in the past. None of that information is current and instead, is etched into your mind as a result of all your life experiences prior to today. Your behaviors, thoughts and beliefs around healing are imbedded in ideas and concepts that are old, rigid and from so many diverse sources from an obsolete time. Our healing consciousness originates from those who raise us, namely parents, family, friends, school teachers, religious institutions, news and now social media. That was then and this is now. Everything changes including the way we become ill and heal, nothing remains the same. You are here in this moment, a different time, a new time, looking forward into the future of your new understanding of what illness is and how you *know* that healing takes place or not. Not everyone gets this chance or has this opportunity that you do right now to begin reformatting your healing consciousness. While old ideas may seem difficult to change, presented here and based on science is a new paradigm in healing, a new understanding of illness and health from a more expansive, quantum level of understanding, opening doors to the greater possibilities in healing that lie beyond what you have been told in the past and what has been generally accepted by the masses.

The Five Secrets for Healing Yourself and Others will broaden your understanding of illness and healing. It is a theory that unfolded and emerged in my process over decades of observation of patients in clinical practice, in-depth research, and study of therapies and patient outcomes. This included the observation of many thousands of patient visits and their responses to a multitude of healthcare procedures and methods not only in my practice but of other physicians and specialists throughout the country. I have had the opportunity to corroborate findings with patients who have undergone treatment by most every healing modality.

In life versus the laboratory, healing can take place in all different ways or fail to transpire. A body might respond to any number of treatments, from taking medication, having chiropractic care to nutrition, acupuncture, surgery, homeopathy, sound therapy and even crystals to name just a few. A person might also simply spontaneously heal. The reality is that for healing of any kind to take place, whether in Western medicine, Eastern medicine or energy medicine of all types, there are *five essential components for healing* that need to be aligned. *"The Five Essential Secrets to Healing Yourself and Others,"* is found in the alignment of these five essential components. The necessity for the five essential components for healing to be aligned, will be true whether for a cut on a finger, an infection, joint pain and including cancer. Also, to the *extent* that healing takes place and while dependent on several factors, it will always include having these five essential components for healing aligned.

My hope is that this book serves as a knowledge and experiential base for expanding what I call your *Healing Consciousness*, meaning your present knowledge and understanding of illness, along with the way you *believe* healing is supposed to take place. I offer here tools that will improve your ability to support your body and those of others in the healing process.

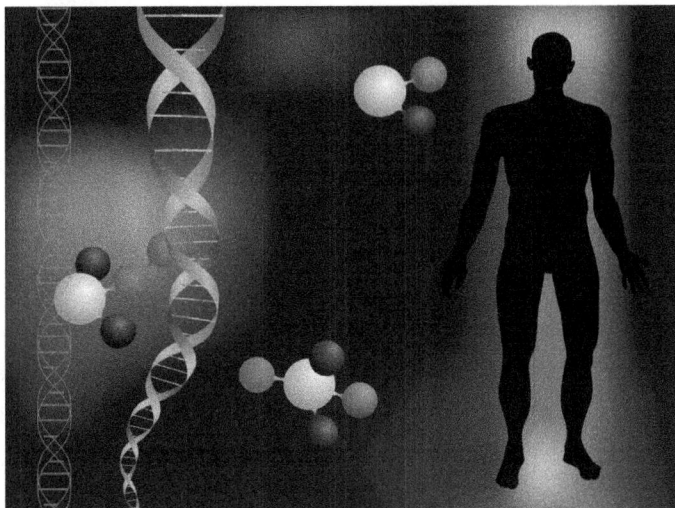

CHAPTER ONE

Re-Evolutions in Healing

As far back as I could remember into my childhood, the first person I had awareness of being sick, was a grandmother from my mother's side of the family. We would visit her in a retirement home when I was about six-years-old and was told she had Parkinson's disease. While I did not understand what that condition was, from that time forward, I found myself wondering why doctors didn't fix her and spending a lot of time pondering all illness and healing. I would ask questions like, why was it that people got sick in the first place, especially if they were taking care of themselves and living healthy lifestyles? Up to that point in my youth, it seemed that anytime family or friends got sick, they improved on their own whether they visited the doctor or not. Somehow, I was sure that the body had some sort of system that automatically healed itself. And if that was the case, I wanted to understand why all disease could not be cured by the natural healing system of body and if not, why advances in science and doctors didn't have all the tools to cure disease. It made no sense to me that people were dying before they were very old. These questions and others around illness and health followed me not only through my youth, but also across my studies in all the sciences, as well as every day of my clinical practice as a chiropractic orthopedist. As a learned practitioner with an ever-growing interest in improving healing and healthcare, my questions and study became more specific. I still wondered though, why it was that with consistent advances in modern medicine and years of research on any disease that not everyone was getting better. More specifically, the question that was most always at the forefront of my mind was, "In a large group of people with the same illness or disease, why was it that they didn't all get better with the same treatment? The treatment that was clinically proven and tested to heal or cure that condition? Some would respond to treatment and others would not. And in the same group of people with the same disease, why was it that any one of them might respond to any one of many dozens of different treatments, but not to the others?"

Another influence on my perspective regarding health was knowing that the grandmother on my father's side of the family had been diagnosed with colon cancer at age forty-five. She was given somewhere between six months and one year to live. To her doctor's dismay, she declined the generally accepted medical treatment of the day. That would have included chemotherapy, radiation and partial removal of her colon. At this time in medicine, both chemotherapy and radiation dosing were yet to be understood and controlled, as was minimizing the radiation of surrounding healthy tissues. In effect, larger areas of body were radiated, not uncommonly resulting in patients dying from radiation poisoning. Instead of undergoing that recommended treatment, she chose an alternative care under the guidance of her chiropractor, Dr. Graves. This would raise a lot of alarm for her doctors, but the family who might have been considered *health nuts* of the day, fully supported her choice of treatment, especially considering she was given such a short amount of time to live. Dr. Graves treated her with an unusually long fast, from what I understand more than thirty days, combined with manual adjustments, acupuncture, mineral spas and loads of vitamins. He then put her on a regiment of specific medicinal juicing and taught them how to eat a health promoting vegan diet which she followed for over twenty years. I remember seeing a photograph of Dr. Graves treating her and other images where she is sitting on a bench being treated with acupuncture in China. She survived this health crisis, living a healthy, active life into her mid-eighties, travelling, writing stories for travel magazines and fully enjoying her family.

I realized then and forever after, not only was there more than one way to treat any specific disease, but that there were scores and scores of diverse types of healthcare modalities and *healing methods* for every type of ailment. Some of these therapies were accepted by the medical community and others were not. In my youth, I was exposed not only to the more typical Western medicine, but also to chiropractic, Eastern medicine, naturopathy, acupuncture, herbalism, homeopathy, and far-out energy types of practices, many of which will be addressed here in the book. Since my first awareness of illness and healthcare, non-traditional healing methods have grown to seemingly uncountable numbers, with vast portions of populations subscribing to these alternative treatments. With varying degrees of acceptance, a large portion of the population are now seeking treatment not only with Western medicine but also Eastern medicine, energy medicine, nutritional remedies, food-based cures, even with hands alone or having crystals waved over the body. While some of these methods seem very far-out, the truth is, they all appear to work with varying degrees of success, on some people, sometimes. None of them work on everyone, even those people who have the same condition where we might see a therapy curing one but not the other. This lack of one hundred percent positive response to treatment includes accepted Western medicine, even with its measure of science and research. Not every person with the same disease responds to allopathic medicine. In part, the intention of this book is to answers the question as to why some people heal and others do not, opening the door to greater possibilities for healing while offering practical tools promoting the healing of ourselves and others.

Diversity of Healing Methods and Modalities

We know that there are an almost endless number of healing methods, all with their own unique procedures and protocols. Each of the healing systems are really trying to do the same thing. They are all attempting to identify what the problem is, in other words diagnose the condition. Next, to have the patient or client understand exactly what their illness is, then clearly communicate what treatment would be prescribed in order to cure, improve or maintain the condition. Each time we treat any ailment, it involves, in some sense, reformatting the patient / recipient's healing consciousness. In other words, guiding them to a clear understanding of their condition, knowing what caused their dis-ease, what the most effective options will be to treat the ailment and what exactly the outcome will be. In not only Western medicine, but any type of healthcare or healing, this takes place in the process of clear and present communication. For this clear and present communication to be effective, the doctor / practitioner needs to be completely focused on the patient without distractions of any kind. They need to ask the right questions (taking a thorough history) and perform a focused, specific examination or assessment of the condition based on the patient's history. And finally, arrive at a specific diagnosis or impression which allows the practitioner to design the best treatment plan for that condition, unique for this individual patient, followed by effectively employing the appropriate treatment.

In Western medicine, most doctors believe it is their job to examine, maintain or improve health through a very specific set of protocols. Sometimes these protocols are quite narrow, resulting in treatment that is typically in the form of pharmaceutical substances or surgery. Not uncommonly treatment might be in the form of *observational therapy*, meaning just watching the patient's signs and symptoms until the condition has deteriorated to the point of needing more drastic and urgent pharmaceutical or surgical measures. Dating back more than 2,500 years, Eastern medicine views health as an expression of balance of body, mind and spirit; the yin and yang or balance. Through specific sets of protocols, these practitioners look for patterns of disharmony in systems and organs, with treatment focusing on re-balancing the body through procedures in the form of acupuncture, teas, herbal medicine, massage, exercise (Qigong, Tai Chi) and diet.

In other forms of healing, two-hundred-year-old *homeopathy* is a practice of administering a very dilute dose of the substance causing the disease, thereby triggering the immune system to be activated, creating a defense against the pathogen and ultimately a cure to the condition. As an example, someone with Hay fever, an allergy to grass pollen, instead of taking prescription medication to suppress the symptoms, a homeopathic remedy would be taken in the form of a micro dose of grass pollen. The intention of ingesting this low dose of the allergen, like a vaccine, is to trigger the body's defense system, inducing an increase of antihistamines, boosting white blood cell production and enzymes that would rid the allergens. One of the most prevalent of energy healing practices is probably *Reiki*, a method of channeling *life force energy* (Qi) through the practitioner, out their hands and into the recipient. *Sound Healing* is another form of energy healing quickly becoming popular. This is a method intended to move the molecules and atoms within the tissues of the body, thereby stimulating the natural properties of the body's healing mechanisms. After thousands of years, *acupuncture* has gained mainstream medical acceptance. That acknowledgement by conventional medicine is specifically for pain control while acupuncturist believe that all ill-health can be treated through balancing energy meridians with acupuncture needles or cupping. Changing health through nutrition has been a long-standing healing method, used since the beginning of time, including the 5,000-year-old *Ayurvedic medicine* which combines herbs and minerals. Even *meditation* alone has also been used as a healing practice for many centuries.

In addition to the methods mentioned above are other healing practices treating illness, such as, sound healing employing singing bowls, healing touch, laying-on of hands methods, psychic healing with the power of the mind, aroma therapy treating people using essential oils, color healing, sweat lodges, crystal healing, hypnotherapy, herbal compounds, minerals of Ayurveda, tapping, Shamanism, reflexology, yoga, Qigong and Tai Chi, among many hundreds of other practices. And while any of these healing practices might be considered quackery by conventional medical standards, the fact remains that some people improve and even completely heal from treatment by these methods, even after having failed to respond to scientifically accepted medical practices and procedures.

While modern medical science has infiltrated most all countries around the world, most cultures have historically maintained their own unique holistic or healing practices. Many healing techniques stem from mythology, others from a relationship with nature, spirituality or religious rituals that have been passed down through generations over hundreds or even thousands of years.

Following thirty years of clinical practice while secretly healing patients for fear that I would lose credibility and my referral network of medical specialists, while at the same time retaining more than forty years of healing experience and practice in many forms including study and research, I finally began setting BioCognitive Healing to paper. This new science in healing, based on the premise that the energy of thoughts when guided in a specific manner, in addition to alignment of the five essential components for healing, stimulates the body's natural ability to heal itself. In that process of developing BioCognitive Healing, I began attending every type of healing seminar or course I could find, in order to see what was being taught and practiced. I wanted to know whether there were any methods like what I had been secretly practicing in BioCognitive Healing and to observe how they were being presented. The bad news was, there was nothing being taught similar to BioCognitive Healing. I found no teachings presenting greater possibilities in healing or specific knowledge and understanding of how the energy of thoughts change biochemistry. That was also the good news. I was clear the time had come to let the BioCognitive Healing cat out of the bag, and to work towards reformatting people's healing consciousness with this new paradigm in health and well-being.

Throughout my time of study and research in healing, I was attending every possible related course I discovered. If a healing program was discussed between friends and colleagues, or if a promotion came through my email or in social media and I was available, I would be heading to a new course of some sort, no matter where it would be taking place and whether or not I had any concrete knowledge about what the healing method might have to offer. I studied and experienced so many different methods of healing, including the some of the most popular, such as Reiki, along with other more obscure techniques including, energy healing, sound healing, tapping, healing touch, chakra healing, qigong, polarity therapy and The Reconnection. In that process, I became certified in some of what might be considered the kookiest healing methods. I additionally became certified in hypnotherapy and as an instructor in Qigong Healing Form. Even with all of these, I knew I had only nicked the surface of healing practices.

Each of these healing methods all involved their own set of pro-cedures and protocols. Some methods were as simple as getting quiet in some form (meditating) and doing nothing but allowing the *life force* energies (qi by many names) to flow through your body. Several of the methods, channeled energy through the body of the practitioner to the recipient, while others were bal-ancing energy fields or chakras while including the use of herbal or natural substances. Where one method might be complicated, passing on ancient secret chants, body movements or prayers, another was diagnosing a condition by evaluating the recipient's pulse, leading to the creation of a distinctive medicinal tea. Some systems had been passed down for centuries or millennia, others were more contemporary or even futuristic concepts channeled from non-physical entities. One method claimed to have been brought from another planet! With some techniques, hands were waved over the body around the diseased area or placing hands directly on the body parts involved. Others manipulated energy between the practitioner and recipient. There are an almost endless number of healing methods and practices.

The bottom line is that they were all trying to accomplish the same thing. Whether Western medicine, Eastern medicine or energy medicine, they all wanted to alter the body's biochemistry on a cellular and quantum level. Each method is striving to alter our anatomy and physiology, to move our thoughts feelings and emotions towards a place of understanding, a place of absolutely knowing that we will heal, stimulating the healing mechanisms in the body on a cellular, emotional and energetic level. The primary focus of this book, reveals how aligning the five essential components for healing, bringing us to that place of knowing we will heal, in turn, stimulates the body's natural ability to heal itself.

When I first started attending these healing programs, I was coming with the same question I had been asking for decades, "Why is it that in a large group of people with the same condition, not everyone responds to the same treatment?" And in that same group of people, "Why was it that any one of them might respond to one of many dozens of therapies but not to any of the others?" In attending these courses, I quickly found a better question to be asking. I was seeing some people get better with almost any of these different methods. Clearly not everyone healed, but people were responding in varying degrees who had not been improving with the traditional Western medical model or other healing practices.

The better question I began asking was: "When people responded to a particular method of treatment, what did they all have in common? What was the common denominator in their healing?"

In other words, what did various treatments and healing modalities have in common when someone responded to their treatment? Whether remission, recovery or complete healing being the result of by-the-book medical protocol, alternative treatments, energy medicine, herbs, chants, rituals, diet or simply spontaneous (of unknown origin) healing, what was the key component that all the methods shared? Seeing so many patients and healing recipients with the same conditions, not all of them responding to any one treatment or therapy, but any of them improving with one of the multitude of methods, I soon realized that it was not *what the different methods of treatment had in common* that affected a person's response to treatment. My question changed again. The new question became, "When someone responds to a treatment of any kind, what was it that the individuals themselves have in common?"

This was the key. There was a common denominator shared by each individual when they responded to any one of the various forms of healthcare or healing. No matter the condition, there was something clearly within the person, an aspect that each of them shared when healing from any modality. What I realized, was whether a person responded to a treatment or not directly correlated to their state of mind around illness and health. I call this aspect of conscious thinking, *healing consciousness*. I noticed that whenever someone improved with a treatment, whether in clinical practice or through some sort of healing method, they were all in a similar aligned state of healing consciousness. I would later come to realize that state of healing consciousness as alignment of the five essential components for healing. The reality was that in all these methods, even when they might seem silly or of little consequence, people were getting better. The state of their healing consciousness was the common denominator. And the truth is that they all worked, to varying degrees, on some people, sometimes. This is a major key when expanding our understanding of illness and healing, that *most any method of healing works, to varying degrees, on some people, sometimes.* And the same is true for Western medicine and Eastern medicine as well.

None of the modalities work one hundred percent of the time or there would only be one method of treating any disease. There would have been no need for other forms of treatment to have evolved or remained in use over scores of centuries. This applies just as well to Western medicine. It was clear to me, that everyone healing from any method, had been brought to a similar specific, highly focused, and highly energized state of healing consciousness.

Over next four years, I sat in all these different healing programs, taking notes, observing, keeping journals, participating and talking with the people who responded to treatment. During this process, five specific attributes of people experiencing healing kept showing up in the pages of my journals. Five consistent features in each person who responded to any form of treatment. Through this process, I realized that even in all my years of clinical practice these same features were also present when patients responded to my prescribed treatments. I was fully appreciating the significance of these five essential components for healing, in that to the degree they aligned or not was a major factor in healing and illness. It seemed as if alignment of the five essential components for healing might be an even greater factor in response to treatment than the tangible treatment itself. That to the degree these essential components were aligned, would determine the degree and permanence of healing.

At that point in my studies and following over forty years of experience in healthcare, treating patients, healing, study, research and sitting in these healing programs, I dissected out, defined and refined the five essential components for healing. These five essential components are one of the primary keys for any healing to take place. They are also part of my practice and teaching in BioCognitive Healing. Aligning the five essential components for healing is part of the process for expanding healing consciousness and creating greater possibilities in healing for oneself and others.

While each of the five components for healing are not in themselves so mysterious, the secret lies in the extraordinary influence on healing by alignment of these five essential components. Consciously or unconsciously, every physician, every alternative care practitioner and healing practitioner is already in some way, to varying degrees, trying to align these five essential components required for healing. But far too often practitioners only address one or two of the components, resulting in either lack of response or partial and temporary improvement. Alignment of the five essential components for healing is also responsible for creating vast numbers of accidental or spontaneous healing. Whether within professional practices, energy practices and even in the populations at large who have little or no understanding of the process, accidental alignment of the five essential components for healing is quite common. As practitioners, having a firm understanding of this concept can greatly improve patient / client outcomes. Let us now look at the five essential components for healing.

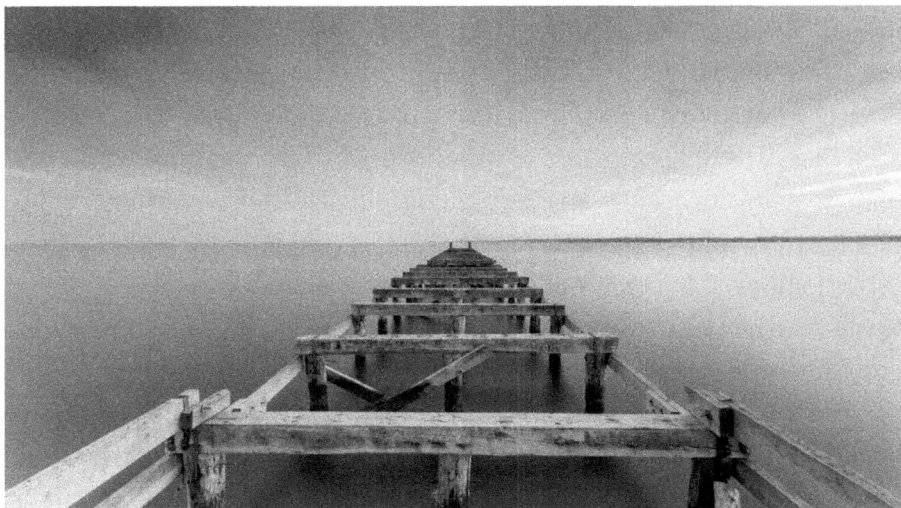

CHAPTER TWO

The Five Essential Components For Healing

Building Blocks for the Secret to Healing

Healing is based on numerous key factors, some are simple to understand through time tested medical procedure and protocol while others are more empirical, logical and inferential, though can still be based on science. Key factors effecting healing in relation to standard medical procedure and protocol include an individual's unique anatomy and physiology. No one injures or heals in the same manner, even if they suffer from the same condition or have the same diagnosis. Imagine two different people with a herniated disc. There are dozens of different possibilities in the way a disc injures at any level and can then be complicated by the varying shapes of joints, age of the tissues, the amount of previous wear and tear of those joints, old injuries, occupational stresses to the local tissues, the quality of the bone (osteoporosis or osteopenia) and other underlying illnesses. Additional factors in the way tissues injure or heal include the cause of the condition, the specific diagnosis, each person's age, heredity, the length of time the damage or condition has been present. Other key factors involve the integrity of the individual's biochemical function, coexisting disease, whether they have undergone treatment and if the treatment was correct for their condition.

Over many decades we have subscribed to a system of healthcare based on scientific protocols and procedure that can seem quite complicated. But as you will see, one of the most important and dynamic factors for healing includes alignment of the five essential components for healing. To the degree that the five essential components for healing are present and aligned will determine the degree, speed, effectiveness and permanence of healing. In my practice of BioCognitive Healing, a method that combines physical science and healing science, reformats healing consciousness, guides precise energy of thoughts in triggering specific tissues and healing systems in the body, along with aligning the five essential components for healing. This alignment of the five essential components is not only a key step in BioCognitive Healing, but always an essential part of healing in every type of healthcare practice.

Following here, I will first present simple book definitions for each of the five secrets for healing yourself and others. Following these definitions, I will break down each of the five essential components separately, as to their deeper importance in relation to how they affect healing, followed by their relationship to one another, and lastly how their alignment is essential in stimulating the body's natural healing capability. None of the five essential components alone carry the power to heal.

1. Knowledge: Thoughts, information, facts, descriptions and skills acquired by a person through experience or education;
   A theoretical or practical grasp of a subject.
   And just to be clear, because we have knowledge on a subject, doesn't necessarily mean it is true or accurate.

2. Understanding: The ability to comprehend.
   Having insight.
   An individual's judgement or perception of a situation.
   Again, because we have an understanding, doesn't necessarily mean this understanding is true or accurate.

3. Belief: An acceptance that something exists or is true.
   Trust, faith or confidence in something or someone.

4. Faith: Complete trust or confidence in someone or something with or without proof. Meaning we unconditionally believe what we are told on any subject. A strongly held belief or theory.

5. Non-attachment to Outcome: Releasing all thoughts, feelings and emotions, related to the outcome of healing, and knowing that there is a reason or purpose for what is happening in one's life.

Now I will begin breaking down each of these five essential components for healing one at a time, in order that you gain a deeper understanding for their importance in healing. Beginning in order as listed, I will start with *knowledge*. When I am referring to knowledge in relation to healing, I don't mean that everyone needs to know all the anatomical, physiological, pathophysiology and medical information for a condition, along with what the appropriate medical procedures and protocols are for treating that condition. Though currently, as intelligent, curious and analytical beings, we are constantly searching the internet for information especially related to our health. This makes it highly important that we filter out inaccurate, biased, manipulated or unhelpful information. Finding correct and helpful knowledge related to a disease or condition is the goal. Unfortunately, the Internet is a place where equal or greater volumes of inaccurate and misinformation exist while easily appearing to be true. Particularly relating to health issues. As you will see, the most helpful knowledge for healing is a very specific kind of knowledge focused on promoting wellness and healing in the body. This specific knowledge will be concisely addressed and involves the reformatting of our healing consciousness, a fundamental intention of this book.

What is knowledge and how is it related to illness and healing?

"Knowledge is Power."

FRANCIS BACON, 16ᵀᴴ CENTURY ENGLISH PHILOSOPHER AND SCIENTIST.

Knowledge:

The origin for the concept of knowledge is said to have come from the word *yada* in the Old Testament, often translated to, *to know*. The problem was that the same word was used throughout the Old Testament with hundreds of other meanings and interpretations than simply, to know. Later, Plato in the 4th century BCE defined knowledge as "justified, true belief." A thousand years later, the 14th century brought the word knowledge into a more contemporary definition as, "a capacity for forming an information base and understanding." *Jna*, a Sanskrit word, identifies knowledge simply and directly, meaning "to perceive or understand." Knowledge is information that we directly perceive and interpret through learning or experience and in our own, unique way. This means that the same knowledge is often interpreted differently by different people. Here is an example, think about a room full of students receiving the same lesson who then join for discussion afterwards. Whether a subject even as factual as mathematics or as theoretical as music and philosophy, there are always many, even dozens of different perceptions or interpretations for the meaning of the lesson. Yet whatever our personal interpretation and understanding might be on a given subject, it becomes etched into our minds, forever considered to be factual knowledge and truth, even though our understanding might differ from others who were in the same lesson. We store our own interpretation as truth regardless of its accuracy. Once we have learned something, accepted that bit of knowledge and stored it as an indelible fact, we may forever defend it as truth even to bitter ends. Irrational, baseless knowledge one might consider as truth, will often be firmly held as legitimate even in the face of clear opposing evidence.

Knowledge we amass and tightly hold onto, originates from many aspects of our lives. Some knowledge develops organically from exposure to people, situations and environments, while other knowledge is formed systematically through what we hear and see from people, media, social media, learning and educational study. Forming knowledge includes the association of previous under-lying, fixed knowledge and life experiences. Knowledge may be philosophical, theoretical, scientific or random. In simple terms, knowledge is the result of anything we see, hear, learn or experience and will be stored either in the conscious or subconscious mind.

The majority of what we consider *true knowledge* arises to a greater percentage out of what we visually see versus what we hear through verbal/auditory transmission, as in, "seeing is believing," or "actions speak louder than words." Information resulting from the act of *observing* (seeing) is easier for the brain to process and requir-ing less interpretation than from what we hear (listening). When we listen to others speaking, or say, hearing a lecture, not only are we listening to that information, but we are creating order to what is being said with our own unique perspective for meaning and truth. You may have noticed that if you watch a television program with the sound turned off, you have a completely different perspective on the quality of the performances and meaning of the story as com-pared to when the sound is turned on. Our visual interpretations carry more weight than do our verbal and auditory cues.

To create a clearer perspective for the idea of knowledge and better understand its relationship to healing consciousness, think of knowledge in the same manner as *data* being entered into a computer. The brain in this example being the computer. Specifically, or randomly, this data as knowledge will enter our brains, often permanently etched there and employed as truthful, accurate information to live our lives by. In this computer comparison, you might imagine stored knowledge in the same way you understand data in the form of words or paragraphs being typed onto the computer, permanently burning them into the hard drive. On their own, words, thoughts and ideas sit dormant and meaningless in the brain as numbers and symbols are stored without meaning on the computer hard drive. The words and images on a computer screen have no effect on the computer, just as words and ideas stored in our minds have no effect on our brain. For there to be meaning of idle data in a computer or in the same manner within a human brain, those words and paragraphs need to be viewed and interpreted by an individual who gives them value and meaning. In the same manner, the words and paragraphs being stored in our brains as knowledge, only have the perspective and meaning that we uniquely give them. In that way, what is important to understand is that our higher conscious-selves can attach interpretations and meaning to the thoughts and words we store in our brains. Someone else might choose a different meaning for the same words and paragraphs stored in their brains. For this reason, and in order to reformat and expand our healing consciousness, it is essential to understand that knowledge stored in our mind especially regarding illness and health, may not always be accurate or beneficial in healing.

Here is a simple example of how we gain and store indelible knowledge in our minds that may not be true. Imagine as a child, Mom and Dad telling you that an apple is called an orange. Since knowledge is simply agreed upon data, an apple could just as easily have been named orange. For your entire youth prior to entering school you think that an apple is called an orange. Then comes the first day of school. You are at lunch with all your new friends and you say, "Hey, would anyone like a bite of my orange?" All the new friends are looking at you puzzled and tell you, "That is not an orange, it's an apple." You could sit there and argue until blue in the face as we often do when defending what we think are truths, though it will remain that everyone else believes your orange is called an apple. It is only called and understood to be an apple, because there is agreement by most people on the planet that this bit of fruit be called an apple. Just because we have knowledge does not mean that it is always true.

Growing up and throughout our lives we learn and store incredible volumes of information and knowledge/data, not all of which is true. We are especially susceptible to absorbing misinformation and misinterpreting information in those years when we are most vulnerable, from birth through our late teens. In the computer analogy, it would be as if, downloading information from the Internet that seems accurate, when it is unknowingly full of bugs and viruses. In effect, knowledge that we are given in relation to any subject throughout our life may contain bugs, viruses while it is being permanently etched in our minds as truth. This is the case whether we are talking about the meanings of words, concepts and ideas in science, religion, politics, food, relationships and including, especially knowledge about illness and health. Without learning to think for ourselves, without raising our consciousness and expanding our inner growth, we could literally live someone else's life in our thoughts and behaviors. We might mature to think and behave as a clone of those who raised us, regarding our knowledge and understanding about any specific life topic. Here, though, I am specifically referring to our perspective on illness and healing. The good news is, that while we carry fixed, unhelpful limitations in our thinking around health, our conscious mind has the flexibility to comprehend and transform into new more helpful perspectives on healing.

Throughout our lives and especially in our youth as sponges for visual and auditory data, we download very specific information and knowledge/data about illness and health. This knowledge originates from those who raise us, namely parents, relatives, spiritual leaders, teachers, neighbors, our doctors and friends. Typically, in this process we learn and store both information that is useful and accurate, but also a large variety of unhelpful information that in affect become barriers which impede or prevent healing. There is some very specific knowledge that can be highly effective in stimulating healing that will be addressed as we progress through the book. While not always easy, to supercharge and enhance our ability to heal ourselves and others, stimulate more rapid and permanent healing, the practices and exercises revealed in this book will be part of reformatting your healing consciousness. In other words, we will be reducing healing misinformation and barriers in our mind, while broadening our knowledge and perspective on illness and the way we believe healing takes place.

As is the case in my practice of BioCognitive Healing, and true for all practices in healing and healthcare, following, are some of the specific types of knowledge required for healing to take place. This is the knowledge when combined with the other four essential components for healing, generates the secret to triggering the body's natural ability to heal itself.

1. Understanding our unique fixed ideas and obstacles to healing, along with tools and practices for reformatting healing consciousness in order to release those blocks and barriers, expanding new possibilities for healing.
2. Knowledge that what the doctor is telling you is true. In other words, confidence in their knowledge and skills.

3. Knowledge that what you have previously researched, read and been told about illness and healing or related to a specific disorder you are currently dealing with, may not necessarily be true. That there might be other more expansive, even simpler possibilities for healing than what you have been told.

4. An understandable, precise knowledge of your condition or disease, including a name/definitive diagnosis and how it occurred.

5. Having visual images of what the damaged tissues look like in their present state, and how they appear when they are healed and normal. Having these images in our minds from a book or computer, of both the unhealthy and healed tissues or organ on a large scale and at a cellular level, creates a reference point for guiding healing. We use these images in our mind's eye as launching points for guiding the healing energy of our thoughts. In this way, we can trigger the necessary biochemical changes for healing in the body. This effect can be either intentional or inadvertent.

6. In BioCognitive Healing, we also teach the exact nature of the energy of a thought, as a wave and solid particle. This defines and explains the way thoughts can be specifically focused and guided in stimulating the glands, tissues and organs to create healing.

7. Knowledge that the illness, disease or condition *can definitely* heal and return to an improved or completely healthy state.

8. Knowledge that we all play an active role in how our body responds to treatment. That there are tools we can employ to proactively improve or cure illness in ourselves and others.

While knowledge and *understanding* in relation to illness and healing can sometimes be confused as one and the same, they are quite different. Let us now look at the meaning of understanding in relation to the five essential components for healing.

"Knowing is not understanding. There is a significant difference between knowing and understanding; You can know a lot about something and not really understand it."

CHARLES KETTERING, AMERICAN INVENTOR AND BUSINESSMAN

Understanding

The term *Understanding* dates to a 12th – century, Old English term literally meaning "to stand beneath or in the presence of a situation, idea or lesson, the comprehension or grasping of information." There are numerous definitions of understanding, including our ability to have empathy or sympathy for someone, to mentally grasp a situation. Understanding might also refer to having an agreement or harmonious relationship, as in *having an understanding*. All understanding is based on an "agreement" between one or more people, for meanings of words, symbols, knowledge, information, thoughts, ideas and concepts. This agreed understanding for the meaning of words, gives order to the world and allows communication between people.

A most literal way to define how we come to an understanding, is through *our own unique perspective* on what we have learned, seen, been told or experienced. In other words, understanding is our perspective and comprehension of stored knowledge. In the computer analogy, knowledge being all the data downloaded (words and paragraphs) into our minds, understanding would be the result of our ability to render that data meaningful and useful (purposeful perspective). Knowledge and understanding together form the foundation that generates the thoughts and intentions important for healing. Those thoughts trigger physical and anatomical changes in the body, creating illness or healing. And as is the case with knowledge, just because we have an understanding, doesn't mean that it is true or correct.

As an illustration, think for a minute about knowledge and understanding, say, in relation to religion. Each religion includes some type of holy text, like the Bible or Quran. Each book is a filled with agreed upon words and symbols or data, building knowledge, around its unique religious beliefs and rules. These books over many centuries, have all been re-written, re-interpreted and understood in more ways than one. There are countless variations for the understanding of these books. These different understandings for each holy text, have created hundreds of different branches of religion based on earlier versions of the same book. Christianity for example, from an original text rose Catholicism, Protestants, Lutherans and Baptist, to name just a very few. The same is true for the Quran and other holy texts that have gone through a wide variety of interpretations leading to many different versions of the same religion. Think about people who have assorted and diverse understandings of the same written words on any subject. Each person's perspective is based on what they have uniquely seen, heard, learned and experienced during their lives to any one point in time. It is this unique and diverse evolution and variation in understanding that leads to not only large numbers of religions arising out of one original holy text, but of a variety of perspectives on any given subject, including illness and health. This should make it clearer, that whether talking about religion or any other topic, just because we have knowledge and understanding does not mean it is necessarily true. In this book, I am talking specifically about our knowledge and understanding of illness and health. What I most want you to understand here, is that in any knowledge/data about health and illness, there can be a variety of interpretations for how the condition occurred and what the solutions might include. In other words, our information about illness and health, unfortunately even from our doctors, may or may not be accurate or true. One last note here, there are no variations in a proper diagnosis. There are plenty of cases where mis-diagnosis takes place. But a condition is either present with specific signs, symptoms and diagnosis or mis-diagnosed.

To better appreciate how we gain and deeply etch knowledge and understanding into our subconscious minds about illness and health that may not be true, I present the following example: Imagine a time when you are growing up through the impressionable childhood years when primary aspects of your healing consciousness are developing. Think about a time during those formative years when someone in the family got sick. Mom and Dad typically called the doctor. While calling the doctor is probably the proper thing to do, what we learn from that, what becomes etched into our youthful healing consciousness, is that "when we get sick, if we don't call the doctor, we don't get better." But we know this isn't necessarily the case. People can go to the doctor and not get better, while others improve without seeing a doctor. The point here is, that just because we have knowledge and understanding of something, in this case about illness and health, does not mean it has to be true.

Don't get me wrong, when we are talking about illness, I'm not saying you shouldn't call the doctor. What I mean is that greater possibilities are usually present for healing beyond the ones we typically associate with a specific condition. You will understand more as you read through the book, how healing can be initiated from the very first thought of an illness, even potentially be healed prior to getting to medical help. This process takes place through aligning the five essential components for healing and through the energy of our thoughts, specifically triggering the healing systems and tissues in the body, often unconsciously. It always comes back to the way we are thinking. When the five essential components for healing are aligned, the energy of our thoughts are moved to take these actions. Would it not be ideal if you were sick, to arrive for your doctor's appointment healed already, having your doctor tell you that you are fine? This is a surprisingly common occurrence even if we seldom hear about it. How many times have you called the doctor for an appointment and begin to feel better as soon as you hung up the phone? This takes place regularly in every healing and healthcare practice. There is a very powerful mechanism from the energy of our thoughts that stimulate the body's natural ability to heal itself.

Ideally it is becoming clearer, that the way we have understood illness and healing is not necessarily accurate or the only way these processes can unfold. Especially, regarding the effects of health information we were inundated with growing up that may not be true. Realize that this type of information has been affecting both the way we get ill and heal.

In order to enhance your abilities to heal ourselves and others, through aligning the five essential components for healing, based on knowledge and understanding, it is important that the recipient or patient have confidence in the practitioner or doctor. In other words, there needs to be trust that the doctor or practitioner has the knowledge, the understanding of the health issue, in addition to the patient trusting the doctor's diagnosis and recommendations for treatment.

The bottom line is, I want patients/recipients and all healthcare/healing practitioners to know, that along with their current perspective and understanding for a health condition and prospects for treatment most typically within the accepted medical model, there are most often additional possibilities for healing. And I reiterate, I'm not saying don't go to your doctor. It is important to be under the guidance of your doctor, but also, you should be doing everything you possibly can to get well. This might include allied, ancillary and/or alternative healing methods. Think about it, let us say you want to lose weight. You would not just take a pill, solely have bariatric surgery or only exercise. What you would do to most effectively lose weight, would include modifying eating habits, exercise, maybe go to support meetings, meditate, journal, possibly include psychotherapy or groups, breath empowerment practices, smoothies and other alternatives. And the same is true when addressing any disease, illness or injury. Just taking a pill or having surgery is not doing everything possible for the greatest healing outcome. And whatever method of care you choose for any ailment, be sure that you have a practice that includes expanding your state of healing consciousness and the aligning the five essential components for healing.

BioCognitive Healing, the method I practice and teach, is based on the premise that, "thoughts change biochemistry." In other words, our thoughts in their physical and energetic nature, have the capability of triggering the immune system, glands, tissues and organs, in healing or causing disease. A primary feature of this process as with every healing and healthcare modality, requires alignment of the five essential components for healing. These are the six steps in the practice of BioCognitive Healing:

1. Understanding and removing limiting, fixed ideas about illness and healthcare and reformatting healing consciousness, towards greater possibilities in healing.
2. Aligning the five essential components for healing, bringing the recipient to a place of *knowingness* that they will absolutely heal.
3. Having an understanding for the nature of the energy of a thought along with the knowledge that *all physical matter has the same energetic properties*. Then, strengthening and focusing the

physical and energetic nature of the energy of thoughts, in order to guide them in triggering specific glands, tissues, organs and systems within the body's natural healing system.

4. Having images in the recipient's mind, visualizing specific body areas and unique images of their condition, both in the state of illness and in perfect health.

5. Lastly, guiding highly concentrated, focused energy of thoughts to stimulate the involved tissues, glands, organs and cells in triggering the immune system and body's healing mechanisms. This process transforms the cells and tissues from a condition of dis-ease to a state of optimal balance and health.

6. Employing closing affirmations to seal within the body, an ongoing healing process. More information on BioCognitive Healing can be found by visiting my website.

Through alignment of the five essential components for healing, bringing yourself or recipient to a place of knowing without a doubt, within every cell of your body and within the energetic nature of energy you are, that you can and will heal. This is my primary intention for you in reading this.

None of the five essential components for healing carries the power to stimulate effective or permanent healing on their own. Each of them supports and builds on the other, resulting in a compound effect. While knowledge and understanding are the first essential steps necessary in creating healing on the deepest level, they require the foundations of the other three essential components for healing, belief, faith and non-attachment to outcome.

Belief

Belief --- An acceptance that something exists or is true. Trust, faith or confidence in something or someone.

"The world we see that seems so insane is the result of a belief system that is not working. To perceive the world differently, we must be willing to change our belief system, let the past slip away, expand our sense of now and dissolve the fear in our minds."
WILLIAM JAMES, AMERICAN PHILOSOPHER AND SCIENTIST.

There was a time when I believed that the next two components for healing, *belief* and *faith*, were the most important. That people could solely heal from having some sort of *pure* belief and/or faith experience. I thought that spontaneous healing might simply be the result of spiritual faith. But I soon learned otherwise. Based on more than forty years of healing and clinical practice, study and research, it became clear to me that without the other three essential components for healing as a foundation, belief and faith alone always resulted in enormous amounts of *wishing and hoping*.

"Just as no one can be forced into Belief, so no one can be forced into Unbelief."
SIGMUND FREUD, AUSTRIAN NEUROLOGIST AND PSYCHOANALYST.

What Freud is pointing out, is the way we hold steadfastly to our beliefs and that changing a belief is no simple task. He thought a belief was unlikely to be changed simply by learning additional information in the classroom or by being forced in some way to change. Beliefs are deeply ingrained as a result of our early learning, life experience and all that we had seen and heard, especially in our childhood. Altering an old belief or having a new belief is accomplished either through brainwashing or making a conscious choice. A conscious decision to change the way we think, a choice to be receptive to new ideas and new possibilities, will open the door to revising or creating new beliefs containing greater truths. The result can be more expansive, effective truths, growing our life experience and gaining new positive, useful skills in healing.

The idea of *a sense of belief*, dates to ancient Greece in the 6th century BCE, where it was represented by a combination of two words, *pistis and doxa*. Pistis was defined as confidence, conviction or trust. Doxa referred to opinion, probable knowledge or trust in something. The word *belief* itself, evolved around the 12th century. By the 14th century, it had become most often associated with religion, as referring to *trust in God*. In modern times, beliefs are related to our feelings and life view on literally all aspects and subjects in our existence.

We live our lives based on beliefs that are deeply etched in our subconscious mind, making them not always so easy to change. A belief is based on knowledge we have gained, taking that knowledge and creating an understanding as it relates to ourselves and our surroundings. The belief is formed when we fix those understandings and perspectives or judgements in our subconscious mind, establishing *a personal truth* regarding any idea or principle. There are many ways we process knowledge and information, forming specific conclusions of truth for each belief. Unconsciously, we permanently engrave this new knowledge into our minds and will consider it to be true, with or without evidence. There is an enormous emotional attachment to these ideas we have decided to believe to be true. Whether talking about our specific religious beliefs, eating habits or ideas around illness and health. A belief might be held by one person and thought silly by another. Take for example those who *believe* their consciousness will be elevated in the next life by not eating animals. Or an athlete believing there is only one specific regiment of training that will improve their performance. There are those who carry a deep set of beliefs around wearing amulets and lucky charms to perform better or be protected. As you can see, there may be little verifiable proof to support these beliefs and surely as much opposing evidence. Most of the time, we live by our beliefs without even thinking about them. But if one's beliefs are challenged, they are often fought for, even to a bitter end. Religion, diet or sports, people are very attached to their beliefs.

Once we arrive at a specific belief about any subject, we maintain a high bias for that belief, holding fast to these ideas, true or not. Some people are willing to literally die for their beliefs. In the process of developing, justifying and making a judgement for a belief, we then spend significant amounts of time throughout our lives seeking and retaining information that supports our beliefs. Some people spend as much or more, disproving other contradicting beliefs in order to deepen their own. Belief doesn't require true introspection or circumspection. Beliefs can develop intentionally by, say, studying or attending classes on a subject of interest, or unconsciously through learning by the example of family members and friends, especially in our youth. Beliefs are built brick by brick over years, even over lifetimes. Our beliefs create a bias that we strive to constantly prove and maintain.

With strong justification for our beliefs over a lifetime, as true and solid as they may feel, beliefs have arisen from a long and imperfect processes, maintaining an open door to errors in truth. Whether our acquired beliefs are true or untrue, they ultimately guide most every thought, word, action and behavior. Beliefs create our global paradigm, the way we perceive order in the world. From the simplest to the most important and complex thoughts we have and decisions we make, they are all limited or unconstrained, based on our beliefs. Beliefs lead us throughout our lives in making choices, including in life and death situations. Beliefs start and end wars. They are powerful and deeply-seated. Accurate or not, we become very attached to our beliefs. This is the case regarding beliefs about everything, including our careers, types of schooling, the way we raise our children, friends, relationships, our eating and exercise habits, the ways we drink or smoke, sleeping habits and our understanding of science and spirituality. Everything and everyone in our lives are affected by our beliefs. I want you to have a deep understanding for the nature of how and why our beliefs are created so that we can specifically address our limiting beliefs regarding illness and health. This might allow us to alter the way we think, behave and take-action when faced with disease and healing.

In order to enhance our ability to heal ourselves and others, we need to expand our healing consciousness and reformat much of what we have learned about illness and health. One goal, not only in Bio-Cognitive Healing, but ideally in all forms of healthcare, is to remove barriers and limited thinking in relation to the nature of an illness at-hand, understanding that there are many options for care beyond what any single source might be telling us, and also that healing can take place in surprising ways, such as, spontaneously. This process of expanding our healing consciousness, peels away preconceived judgements or beliefs, bringing that part of our minds to a childlike, unadulterated perspective of greater possibilities for healing. A young child with an illness doesn't obsessively think about getting better as is typical for adults. Children are living in the moment, while having a natural unconscious *knowing* or expectation that they will get better, rendering them more susceptible to the therapeutic benefits of a treatment. When children improve from a health condition, they hardly notice because they are so busy and distracted by the trials and joys of life. A concept maybe difficult for some people to understand, is that prior to an infant or young child being filled with narrow, limited beliefs surrounding illness and health, these pure of mind and heart beings still well connected to their spiritual origin, I believe, naturally heal of themselves and their families with the unadulterated energy of their thoughts.

One of the difficulties in attempting to bring our self to a place of profound belief, without the foundation of knowledge and under-standing, would be like trying to build a house from the top down without a foundation. Trying to have a deep belief in something without the knowledge and understanding, would be like me throw-ing you the keys to my car and telling you to take it for a ride, only you have never even seen a car before, — and, it is a manual shifting car.

So here is what might happen in that situation. You take the keys, walk over to the car and sit in the driver's seat. You have no idea how to start the car or even what the key is used for, let alone where to put it. The knowledge and understanding of where you put the key and how to start the car is essential. You need to know and understand that once started, the left foot presses the clutch to the floor while the right foot pushes the accelerator. Once the engine is revved to the proper strength, the shift lever is moved into first gear, while the clutch is slowly released, engaging the transmission in coordination with altering pressure on the gas pedal. At the same time, both hands must be on the steering wheel, which turn the front wheels left and right. Once the car is up to a specific speed, the clutch gets depressed again, while at the same time, letting off the gas pedal, shifting to second gear and slowly releasing the clutch. Plus knowing the right foot is used for braking on the middle pedal along with all the rules and driving codes. The point is, we need a significant amount of knowledge, understanding and practice before we can drive a car. We could not just drive a car based on *believing* we could.

In the same manner, we need a foundation of knowledge and understanding to be able to create a belief about anything, including illness and healing. We know that a car drives, (the belief) we've seen them. But we also know that it cannot be driven without the foundation of knowledge and understanding. The same is true in the case of a religious belief. Unless we are taught through knowledge and have a sincere understanding of that religion, we would lack the necessary belief. There needs to be the underlying groundwork of knowledge and understanding to generate a belief. But again, alone, belief is not enough to create healing.

Someone might say, "Well, what about naïve cultures who have medicine men, shaman or witch doctors? They seem to have some success curing some disease" with no formal schooling and maybe only a simple apprenticeship handed down over generations. It is true, that primitive cultures have been curing disease without any formal schooling or education since the beginning of time, which reminds me of a story, "The Three Hermits" by Leo Tolstoy.

In summation of "The Three Hermits," a Christian Bishop on his way to a monastery in Russia, keeps hearing from the fisherman of Three Hermits on an island who are holy men. These holy men are said to heal people and are working towards saving their own souls. The Bishop wants to see how these three holy men are healing people and asked to be taken to the island. After long travel at sea, he is rowed in a small boat to the island from the ship where he meets the three hermits who are pleased to see him. The Bishop asks them what prayers they use to help others and themselves. The hermits are very happy to tell him, "Three are ye, three are thee, have mercy upon us." The Bishop says no, no, no, those are not proper prayers. He sees them as naïve and wishes to teach them lessons and proper prayers from the Bible, which he does. As it is becoming dark, the Bishop gets back into the row boat to return to the ship. As they row away, the island becomes smaller and smaller until he could no longer see the hermits at the shore. Barely able to see the island anymore, the Bishop suddenly noticed a glimmering light coming closer and closer from that direction at a quickened pace. Difficult to make out what it was, he soon realized it was the three hermits running hand in hand atop the sea as if it were dry land. Reaching the Bishop in the boat, they kept repeating, "We forgot your teaching, servant of God, teach us again!" The Bishop leaned towards them, told the Hermits to continue with their own prayers and that it was not for him to teach them.

There are three relevant points to this story, the first being the way we form fixed beliefs that may or may not be true. And at least may or may not be true for everyone. The Bishop had a set of beliefs regarding proper prayers for connecting with God. In the same manner, the three hermits had their own set of beliefs about prayers. Each of which could be equally valid and true for one but not the other. The second point is that while it might seem that the hermits were creating miracles based on blind, naïve belief and faith, the reality is that they would have had some type of underlying knowledge and understanding. Their knowledge and understanding might be as simple as knowing that the ritual of saying their prayer in a certain way, in a certain place or time and knowing that this ritual would cause changes in people's minds and bodies. The hermits had their own unique set of learned knowledge and understanding underlying their belief and faith. There will always be a foundation of knowledge and understanding supporting belief and faith. The third feature of this story is that the hermits were lacking the preconceived judgements and limiting barriers in thinking inherent in the Bishop, regarding how healing is supposed to take place. The Bishop's knowledge and culture, created fixed beliefs, limiting his ability to heal in the way the three hermits were doing. Their childlike purity of mind remained, without all the learned limitations and mental barriers in relation to illness and health. The bottom line is that belief and faith alone are not enough for most people to expand or develop their healing consciousness, in a way that creates powerful healing for themselves and others. Spontaneous healing, which is quite common, never takes place through belief and faith alone.

And there are other problems with belief and faith. First, they both have religious connotations which turns-off some people, thinking that *healing* is some sort of religious ritual. On the other hand, people following a specific religion might feel uncomfortable if they *thought* a healing process involved reference to something ungodly, involving unsuitable pagan rituals of a sort. An atheist may find talking about belief and faith to be religious, distracting them from opportunities in healing. To be clear, healing is not a religious event. It may be helpful to understand that there are many types of belief, some related to spirituality or religion and others that are not. For our purposes, let us look at two types of belief, "Belief-in" someone or something and "belief that" an idea or something exists or is true. Belief-*in*, is most commonly associated with religious devotion to God or some higher power typically without proof or evidence. Belief *that* something exists or is true, refers to believing, say, a scientific experiment, social or environmental theory is true and accurate. With this understanding, removing the idea of belief in healing from any religious attachment, I will point out that spirituality (hopefully present in religion though not necessary) does have the ability to enhance and compound the effects of a healing practice. This point will be addressed shortly.

The following two concepts might better explain the type of healing I'm referring to that is not based on religion or spirituality. The belief that is optimally present for healing would consist of:

1. Confidence and trust based on accurate knowledge and understanding that healing will without a doubt take place even beyond what you may have learned in the past.
2. Belief that healing can take place in many unexpected ways, based on physical and metaphysical science, leading to more expansive truths about the nature of illness and healing.

Faith

Complete trust or confidence in someone
or something without proof.
A strongly held belief or theory.

*"Faith consists in believing when it is beyond
the power of reason to believe."*

VOLTAIRE, FRENCH PHILOSOPHER, HISTORIAN, AUTHOR.

Faith can occur in the form of an innate feeling, trust or confidence in someone or something, or be based on a distinct set of information. As is true for any *word*, faith is a symbol representing a commonly agreed upon definition. As a feeling, faith is a primitive, reverential experience of confidence and trust. In its simplest form, the word faith dates to early 13th century Middle English, feith, via the Latin word *fidem*, meaning *trust*. You have probably heard the expression, "a leap of faith." This refers to jumping into a situation, solely based on a feeling of truth, or resulting from what someone else told us to believe, even if lacking logic or common sense. When you think about it, faith is largely irrational in that it is hard to explain and most often accompanied by a lack of interest in examining its credibility. But the feeling of faith runs so deep that it becomes personally indisputable, whereby it will be defended even to a bitter end. Most often, people associate faith with religion, as with *faith in God* or a higher power of some sort. Religious faith is largely derived through blind acceptance of teachings that may lack rationality or common sense, creating obedience to an authority. Faith can sometimes involve a process of fooling ourselves into thinking that we lack the logic necessary to validate an idea with proof in order to support a belief. Even in *atheism* faith is even present. Understand that having faith is not exclusive to religion or spirituality.

Non-religious faith can be present in science, in politics, views on the economy and of course, be related to illness and healing. In science, a theory or hypothesis are unexplainable beliefs, sometimes considered laws of physics even if they are yet to be proven. Students of science are not always asked to prove some laws of nature or mathematics they might employ in their study and research. They take many principles as certainty, applying them in research, while having faith that truth and certainty will be revealed. Scientists must have faith in themselves, in established laws of physics or in their theories while having no proof. For some examples of non-religious faith, we might look at Thomas Edison. He made more than 1,000 attempts at creating the lightbulb before he was successful. He could have easily given up after two or three failed attempts. What kept him striving for a specific result, rather than giving up, was faith in his theory and commitment to what he believed to be true. Ludwig von Beethoven composed nine symphonies, seven of them after he had become completely deaf. What would have him think he could still compose music when he could no longer hear and fine tune the sounds? Or Michael Jordan being cut from his high school basketball team. Why would he ever think he could be a player in the NBA, especially, becoming the greatest of all time? We might have faith in a politician though we do not really know who they are or how they will affect our country. Or faith in the direction of the economy, while having little understanding of major factors such as the gross domestic product (GDP) or the difference between a budget deficit and the national debt. Faith in all forms are embedded into our minds in the same manner, moving people to continue to believe in something without good reason when at the same time, others may have given up. The important concept to understand here, is that we have the capability of creating and maintaining that same faith when confronted with issues of illness and healing. Whether or not we incorporate spirituality or religion, we can develop strong faith and belief as part of the five essential components for healing, knowing that we will get better.

The biggest problem with the idea of faith alone effecting healing, comes from it being established on trust or confidence without proof, faith is completely blind. In other words, there is no reason or foundation to support having faith. It is easy to think or say that we have faith in someone or something. But subconsciously, our worldview, the culmination of all that we have learned, seen and heard throughout our lives, might instead be telling us that our faith is not truly authentic. Instead, faith might be thought of as an unfounded concept we *try* to hold onto or maintain because *we think we should* have faith in someone or something. We might think we have faith solely based on the habit of telling ourselves we do. But the nature of unjustified or irrational faith that healing will take place, can easily be subconsciously misaligned with how we truly feel and instead turn into *wishing and hoping*. In the process of working with patients and recipients in all forms of healing and healthcare, a natural part of patient management includes a reformatting of the way faith and belief are embedded in our minds around the ideas of illness and health. And just to be clear, faith is important, but alone is not enough to generate true and permanent healing.

The faith we want to achieve for healing is not religious, nor does it have to be related to spirituality. We want to develop faith as;

> Complete and total trust without blocks or limited thinking, based on knowledge, understanding and belief that without question, healing will take place.

Developing this type of faith is not always easy to achieve or maintain in the face of a serious illness such as cancer that may have been determined to be fatal. But remember, most of us know or have heard of someone like my grandmother, who was given weeks or months to live but who instead survived and thrived for many years, spanning even a full and productive life. In the same token, we have heard of those who were diagnosed with early, mild forms of cancer which are almost always curable, when instead these patients died within days or weeks of the diagnosis. The point being, that just because we're are given a diagnosis and prognosis, does not mean illness or healing can only take place in that one way. That even having been told we have a progressive condition, I'm saying there is always a possibility for remission or complete healing. An example of this would be Stephen Hawking, the theoretical physicist and cosmologist from Cambridge University in Great Britain. He was diagnosed at age twenty-one, with amyotrophic lateral sclerosis (ALS), also known as Lou Gehrig's disease. ALS is a progressive neuro-degenerative disease that has a typical mortality rate of two to five years from the diagnosis. Not only did Stephen Hawking not die by age twenty-six, but he lived to seventy-six years old, and in that time changed the world view in physics and cosmology. Even in the face of what might seem to be insurmountable odds, there is always good reason to maintain faith based on knowledge, understanding and knowing there are unknown possibilities for healing.

Retaining faith at times takes practice. When we have those feelings of doubt, the blocks and limitations of our healing consciousness, it is necessary to revisit the knowledge and understanding of greater possibilities for healing and exercise non-attachment to outcome. We need to be able to release old ideas about illness for how any condition is *supposed to heal*, be an active participant in treatment and in modifying our healing consciousness to the greater truths and possibilities in healing. In other words, letting go of the old thinking that serves no helpful purpose and allowing it to be okay that an illness can heal in ways we never thought possible.

Ultimately, it is important to build faith through new knowledge and understanding as one of the five essential components for healing. This process includes creating total trust that healing will take place, and I refer you back to the section on having knowledge and understanding. Another factor for building faith, is in gaining confidence in our physician or practitioner, their knowledge and their ability to clearly communicate details of treatment and healing. The tools included in this book for aligning the five secrets for healing, are designed to expand healing consciousness, while building and maintaining each of the essential components.

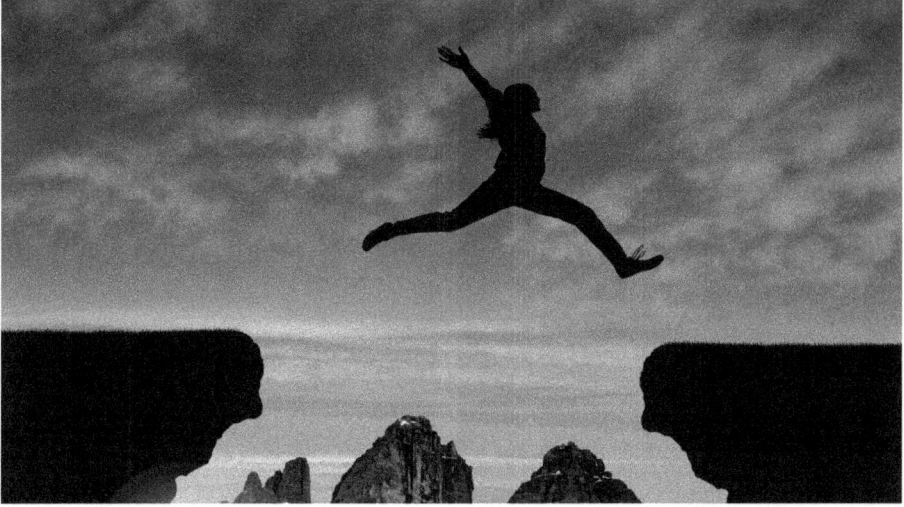

CHAPTER THREE

Non-Attachment To Outcome

To this point, I have covered the first four of the five secrets to healing yourself and others: *knowledge, understanding, belief* and *faith*. The fifth essential component, *non-attachment to outcome*, should not be diminished because it is being addressed last, as it carries equal weight to the other four components for healing. They all need to be present and aligned. This fifth component for healing will be the final, though by all means essential force in aligning the thoughts, emotions, anatomy and physiology in healing. This alignment will result in the unrestricted triggering of processes in our biochemical makeup that activate the body's innate healing abilities, as well as a consolidating a powerful state of healing consciousness.

To recap the effects on our healing consciousness by the first four essential components and to better understand this new paradigm of healing, first remember that because we already have some knowledge, understanding, belief and faith related to illness and healing, it may not be accurate or true. It is important to realize we have the ability, to reformat those inaccurate limiting beliefs, replacing them with truer and more expansive possibilities in healing. We now understand how knowledge is simply data that has been downloaded into our cerebral consciousness computer. Also, we recognize understanding, as our personal unique perspective of that data/knowledge, realizing this knowledge and understanding is based on a broad set of set life experiences. The source of those life experiences and learning comes from an incalculable number of individuals and sources, each with their own unique bias based on their personal life experiences. The result being, that from a very young age, our knowledge, understanding, belief and faith deeply fixed in our subconscious mind, can in-fact be, someone else's life perspective, with all *their* built-in limitations and inaccuracies. If we live unaware from subconscious, ingrained and inaccurate truths related to illness and health, we might follow mis-guided beliefs to unproductive or undesirable outcomes in healing. In this chapter I address the fifth essential component for healing, *non-attachment to outcome.*

What is non-attachment to outcome? I have students attending retreats who often say, "Why should I not be attached to getting better? Why would I not want to constantly be thinking about getting better, wanting to be well, desiring a positive outcome and thinking optimistically about a health condition?" While it might seem intuitive to be habitually thinking in positive ways about health issues, too much focus and attention on health concerns can have an opposite effect. In other words, having too frequent a focus, of even positive thoughts, can just as likely inhibit, slow or even prevent healing. While important to always do everything we can regarding our health and healing, it is also vital that we avoid becoming obsessively attached to the outcome, and here is why.

We now know every thought alters our biochemistry and physiology in either positive or negative ways. This creates problem with being attached to outcome if we are constantly thinking about wanting a disease or health issue to get better. Constant awareness of a condition keeps regular, ongoing thoughts of illness at the forefront of our minds. Those relentless thoughts, consciously or not, will lead to opposite feelings and ideas. In other words, there are equivalent thoughts that the illness may get worse. Obsessively thinking about healing and having thoughts of a progressive worsening of an illness go hand in hand. The effect of being attached to outcome, thinking at times an illness is getting better and other times that it is getting worse, creates a healing consciousness of *wishing and hoping* improvement with take place. The desired goal is instead, a state of *knowing* without a doubt that healing will occur.

This theory of non-attachment to outcome is not new and is present in early Buddhist philosophies. Late 18th —century physicians including William Falconer in 1788, recommended what he called a therapeutic procedure of *redirecting the mind.* His theory was that if the patient's mind is redirected away from their condition, it would eliminate illness thoughts and symptoms. In turn, this would allow them to get better. He prescribed procedures that prevented the patient from dwelling on their condition, recommending "thoroughly occupying the patient's mind, leaving no room for recollection or apprehension of the disorder." He realized that patients obsessing about their condition responded poorly to treatment. During this period in the late 18th century, while distracting the patient's thoughts from their condition, Dr. Falconer used placebo pills in the form of bread crumbs coated with silver leaf to boost the patient's sense of being properly treated. New research tells us that people who keep "pain diaries," a daily log of how backpain progresses, or in other words, regularly dwell on their condition, responded far less and slower to treatment than those who did not keep a pain diary. Redirecting the mind is also an aspect of hypnosis, meditation and most forms of psychotherapy.

There is a medical diagnosis termed, *illness anxiety disorder* or *somatic symptom disorder*. This terminology has replaced identifying a patient as a *hypochondriac*, due to the negative stigma around this term. Illness anxiety disorder is a serious form of being *attached* to one's illness and treatment outcome. It is specifically a pre-occupation with illness. In this condition, a patient might think they have an illness or will contract another disease which do not already have. The patient amplifies in their mind, symptoms of an illness that are not as clinically significant as they believe. They will obsessively and excessively be checking themselves, making unnecessary doctor visits and not believing negative results of medical tests. This is a state of high anxiety in which the person is consumed and excessively worried about a condition that may not exist. They interpret minor medically insignificant sensations in their body to mean serious illness. This represents an extreme version of attachment to outcome, often leading to real symptoms in the form of pain, weakness or dizziness, and can over time result in real physical illness. But even non-clinical attachment to a health condition, such as "constantly thinking positively about healing," can easily turn into thoughts of wishing and hoping, which also create limitations and barriers to healing.

When we continuously think about a health issue, even when those thoughts are mostly positive, a pattern of obsessive thinking evolves. As if on automatic pilot, without feeling or sincerity, these thoughts become an unending loop of mental toiling around an illness. Eventually, this obsessive type of thinking turns into *what ifs*. What if my condition magically gets better! What if it doesn't get better? What if it gets worse? What if it all-of-a-sudden, it develops into another illness? What if it seems to be getting better, I have one negative thought, and suddenly it takes a turn for the worse again? What if it never gets better? What if I die? What if, what if, what if... This sort of endless loop of obsessive thinking about a health condition will ultimately create barriers and limitations to healing.

Another way to understand this, is that when we are *trying so hard* to force a healing outcome, we are in effect, creating a constant attachment to our illness. Rather than aligning the five essential components for healing, bringing us to that place of knowing we will get better, our thoughts and emotions instead turn into the wishing and hoping we will heal. One of the best ways to practice non-attachment to outcome, is to be sure that at any given time you have done everything you can in relation to your condition. You have seen all your practitioners, follow your home care guidance and apply healing consciousness practices for aligning the five essential components for healing. When all these actions have been undertaken, you are then able to release all thoughts of illness or healing. Then, go on about your life in joy, working, creating, being productive and living life to your fullest capability.

In order to be unattached to any outcome around your health, you want to be fully present to whatever activity you are engaged in. If there is no productive action you can take related to a health condition, the idea is to avoid focusing on or putting energy into thoughts of illness or disease. If you do find yourself spending unproductive, obsessive time with thoughts on physical ailments, or wishing you *might* get better, refocus that attention. Following here is an illustration of a practice for achieving non-attachment to outcome in those situations. Imagine you are sitting at work or home when out of the blue you have a thought about your health condition. Maybe you felt a sensation or pain in your body, or you might have remembered an upcoming doctor's appointment or test. This can trigger all sorts of thoughts, feelings and emotions around your illness or dis-ease. You might start wondering if it is getting better or thinking that maybe it is progressively getting worse. There might be all sorts of thoughts that your ailment may be improving or not or wondering if you are undergoing the right treatment and using the best doctors. Maybe you are thinking that the condition might cause other health issues, whether the medication prescribed is correct or, if the dose of medication is right. You might find yourself questioning the doctor's recom-mendations or whether he is doing everything he can for your condition. Following here is a simple, straightforward practice for bringing your healing consciousness back to that state of *knowing* you will heal, without being attached to the outcome. To break the cycle of obsessive toiling in your mind for whether you are getting better or not, and move your thoughts and body in the direction of healing, take the following actions:

Practice Avoiding Obsessing on Illness

1. At the first thought of your condition, take every possible action you can think of that might move you in the direction of being better. Maybe you need to make that appointment with a doctor that you have been avoiding. Schedule needed tests, take your medicine or vitamins, make a therapeutic smoothie, call your therapist, get up and stretch or exercise. Complete every

positive action you can take towards your healing. When you run out of possible measures you could actively take and there is nothing else you can do;

2. Have one clear, focused, powerfully positive healing thought around your health issue. *Visualize*, in other words, imagine the ailing organ, tissue or system in perfect health and functioning without inflammation or dysfunction. Rather than dwelling on the illness or how you think it might be doing, picture in your mind, the tissues that are dis-eased and see them in a perfectly healed state. Visualize your entire body already healed and in a state of perfect health. Then release all thoughts and focus on the condition.

3. Immediately return to what you were doing prior to having the thought of illness or change what you were doing and take some different actions. Practice being completely present to whatever activity you are involved with in the moment. Your thoughts, feelings and actions should be so filled with your present moment endeavor, there will be no room in your mind for toiling or obsessing about your condition. And, you will be more effective and satisfied about what you're doing in that moment.

These simple steps can break the cycle of obsessive thinking and behaviors around illness and disease, bringing us to that place of non-attachment to outcome. We know that *thoughts change bio-chemistry*. Positive or negative, our thoughts, feelings and emotions trigger chemical processes on both a systemic and cellular level, ultimately altering our genetic coding. With more than 80,000 thoughts a day, we want those thoughts to be positive and healing, while stimulating vitality and joy in our mind and body.

With the fifth essential component, non-attachment to outcome aligned, the five essential components for healing are complete. Not one of the essential components for healing is more important than the other. They are all essential and when aligned, work in concert with each other bringing our healing consciousness to that state of *knowing* that without a doubt, we will heal. This in turn, sets off a coordinated cascade of physiological reactions within the healing systems of our body. The success of all methods of healing, Western medicine, Eastern medicine, all forms of energy medicine and even spontaneous healing, are all the result of achieving that state of knowing that healing will take place. The result of aligning the five secrets for healing taking place either consciously / intentionally or unconsciously will have the same effects of healing. Know that the success of all methods for healing, no matter the procedure, will result when the five essential components for healing are aligned. Achieving this state of healing consciousness is the reason someone from a group of people with the same illness will respond to an unusual or uncommon treatment, while they may have failed to improve with more traditional methods of care. This book is designed to increase your skills at purposefully and intentionally aligning the five essential components for healing, thereby enhancing your innate ability to heal yourself and others.

When the five secrets for healing are aligned, we generate a state of healing consciousness that there is no single word to describe. In this state of healing consciousness, our body becomes highly susceptible to the energetic nature of our thoughts, triggering the immune system, stimulating the glands, tissues and organs necessary to create the biochemical changes associated with healing. While I was looking for a word that best describes the state of healing consciousness, and since I was unable to find that perfect word, I made one up or rather altered a known word to best fit that healing state. The word that best represents that healing state of consciousness when all the five essential components for healing are aligned, is a *Knowingness*.

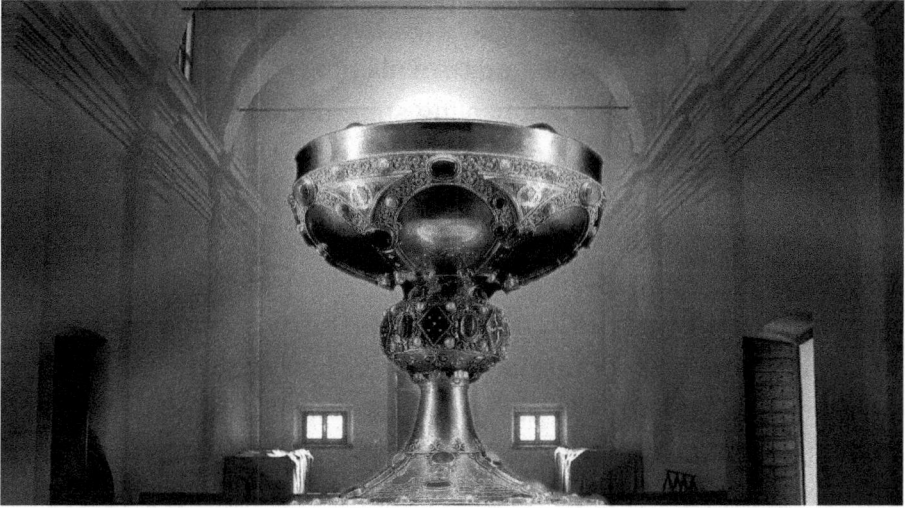

CHAPTER FOUR

Knowingness

Knowingness is an absolute, clear, unwavering, without a doubt "knowing," that healing changes are going to take place. I'm not referring to *just knowing in the mind*, but rather knowing within every fiber of your being, that a condition or illness will be healed. Knowing within ever vibrantly vibrating, energized cell of the body. Knowing within our higher consciousness, within the essence of the greater being of energy we are, beyond the physical body, that without question, without a doubt, complete and definite healing will take place. Because of the importance for expanding our healing consciousness and aligning the five essential components for healing, chapter six is dedicated to explaining tools and practices for achieving and maintaining a healing state of mind. These are practices that compound and enhance the knowledge, understanding, belief, faith and non-attachment to outcome necessary to reformat our healing consciousness, resulting in that all-important state of *knowingness*, that without any doubt we will heal.

Achieving this state of knowingness, is the most important aspect of healing from any condition, disease or injury regardless of treatment method. Coming to this state of knowingness is essential for the fullest and most permanent recovery by any form of treatment. Reaching this place of knowingness is the result of alignment of the five essential components for healing. Anytime we are dealing with an injury, health or medical condition, from the simplest cut on a finger, improving from a surgical procedure, a cold, responding to an antibiotic or even a response to cancer therapy, it is this knowing within the deepest part of our being that will determine the success of treatment. Aligning the five essential components for healing can be more important than the treatments and remedies themselves. It is this knowingness that allows one of dozens of diverse treatments to be effective in healing one person, but not another, even with the same condition.

This process of aligning the five essential components for healing is not only a feature in my practice of Bio-Cognitive Healing, but a primary reason for response to treatment in every form of medicine and healthcare. Whether it is realized or not, every practitioner is following a certain protocol or taking specific steps toward moving a patient or recipient in the direction of broadening their healing consciousness and aligning these essential components for healing. You might wonder, "What about a physician with poor bedside manners, or doctors who are not contentious and thorough in their practice skills and procedures?" To this I would say, just by the nature of choosing a career in medicine or healing arts, besides the clinical aspects of learning and poor bedside manner, there is a natural and ingrained interest by most physicians for helping others. While not always the most effective, this state of the practitioner's healing consciousness moves them by varying degrees in offering their patients some amount of knowledge and understanding for what their condition might be and the options for treatment. In other words, as a result of their interest in health and education, doctors even unknowingly are wanting to alter a patient's healing consciousness in positive directions. Besides educating patients or clients in their condition and treatment, this part of practice procedure is what builds trust in the practitioner. During this process of communicating with their patients/recipients, the expertise and proficiency of each practitioner varies in effectiveness. Some practitioners will be more naturally able to align one or two of essential components, while others might be innately skilled at guiding patients in aligning all five healing components. They may even be generating alignment of the five essential components for healing accidentally, because of their own, already expanded and innate healing consciousness.

The fact is, at times we all innately and often accidentally align the five essential components for healing, thereby healing ourselves and others. Alignment of the five essential components for healing, bringing a patient/client to that place of knowingness, can be the most important process for healing. While every doctor, alternative care practitioner and healer, consciously or unconsciously, are in some way guiding their patients toward this alignment, we all have room to improve our healing skills.

Guiding a patient/recipient to this place of alignment and knowingness results from specific forms of communication and actions when addressing their condition. These methods and actions appear as clinical procedures, protocols and evaluation methods or rituals, such as taking a patient history, performing an examination/assessment or ordering clinical tests. These learned and practiced procedures are the reason even if unconsciously, all practitioners are going to in some way alter a patient's healing consciousness. In every type of practice and through each step of their procedures, it is essential that the practitioner be completely present to the patient/recipient. Being present during communication with the patient is where the greatest share of reformatting healing consciousness is accomplished. To effectively expand healing consciousness and align the five essential components, there can be no distractions for the practitioner or patient. For this to effectively occur, there needs to be absolute presence and engagement between the practitioner and patient/recipient. The goal always being, the patient achieving a state of knowingness, without a doubt, they will heal.

Bringing order to the five essential components for healing will result in seeming miracles of healing. These miracles in healing might include everything from the way a simple cut on a finger repairs itself, to the healing of serious illness that may typically be resistant to treatment and include *spontaneous healing*. This is a good place to address spontaneous healing, which occurs literally every day in various forms within ourselves and those around us. Spontaneous healing can be defined as, "unexpected improvement or disappearance of disease, including for cancer that cannot be attributed to allopathic or Western medicine treatments." While spontaneous healing is often snubbed by mainstream physicians, these practitioners typically have no background in studying this aspect of healing and may have no record for how patients improved or progressed who didn't return to their practices. It is not uncommon that a patient fails to return to their doctor's office because they improved by means that didn't include that physician's services. I believe that most people have either witnessed, heard about or experienced spontaneous healing of some kind.

The US National Library of Medicine, National Center for Biotechnology and The National Institute of Health (NIH), archive all medical research papers, journals, biomedical and life science health data, once only available for physicians, but now accessible to the public. Typing a search for *spontaneous remission*, synonymous for spontaneous healing at the NIH website, reveals a list of over twelve hundred different clinical papers and articles on the subject. These studies include the spontaneous remission not only for common illnesses, but also for a wide variety of rare and fatal diseases. This list of spontaneous remissions in research to name a few, include influenza B infection, lymphoblastic leukemia, Hodgkin's disease, rheumatoid arthritis, kidney disease, Cushing syndrome, breast cancer, endocrine cancer, ulcerative colitis, autoimmune diseases, such as, sarcoidosis, epilepsy and neurological conditions. Realize that the diseases noted in these papers and reports from the NIH don't include the vast number of spontaneous healing that go unreported, detached from clinical research and the healings that take place on daily basis all over the planet without record. In 1993 The Institute of Noetic Sciences in Petaluma, California, created the first database on spontaneous healing. At that time, it included 3500 references from 800 journals in 20 languages and though not current, still provides the largest database of medically *reported cases* of spontaneous remission. This database includes the spontaneous remission from a wide range of incurable, chronic and terminal illnesses, including most types of cancer, including stage 4 malignancies, HIV, cardiovascular illnesses, metabolic disease, diabetes, hypertension and other autoimmune disorders. In the January 2011 Journal of Science, Biology and Medicine, Thomas Jessy, a professor of oral medicine and radiology, reports that after hundreds of years of observation of spontaneous remission of cancer, "it is now accepted as an indisputable fact." He notes that even with the greater standardization and advances in cancer therapy over the last fifty years, patient outcomes are little changed. He remarks, there is almost no change in cancer survival over the last ten years. A recently approved and expensive cancer drug showed only a four month longer survival rate than the patients taking a placebo. It is largely understood that doctors and patients both, overestimate benefits of chemotherapy while underestimating risks and side effects. All these findings point to the fact that spontaneous remission in cancer is not rare.

There currently there are over 2,000 chemotherapy cancer drugs on the market and 5,200 being researched, many of which go public as Independent Public Offerings (IPOs) on the stock market while still being studied. This process of creating a financial windfall for the drug manufacturer by potentially millions of investors, for unproven medicines, may create pressure on researchers that results in biased outcomes. While a large percentage of the population believe that FDA approval of a cancer drug means it is safe and/or effective, this is not the case. The FDA regularly approves drugs to the market that have not proven to cure or help cancer patients live longer. The current environment of prescribing the appropriate dosages for the designated cancer drugs is always an experiment. This is a result of the distinctive nature and unpredictable progression of each cancer, along with the biological uniqueness of every patient. None of these medications are consistently effective in curing any specific cancer, while at the same time damaging other surrounding healthy tissues and systems of the body. Many new cancer drugs approved by the FDA have an annual average prescription cost of $200,000.00 per year. There are cancer medications being marketed at a cost between $374,000.00 and $550,000.00 per dose. Due to poor outcomes in studies, researchers keep lowering the bar for a new drug to be considered successful. The American Society of Clinical Oncology set their goal for new cancer drugs to extend life or control tumor growth for 2.5 months. This is not a very ambitious or consequential goal, while proving true for only one in five medications developed in the last twelve years. We also know that some of the diagnostic and therapeutic procedures for cancer, especially the ones that included chemotherapy and radiation, such as, mammogram, x-ray and CAT scan, can be the cause of, or aggravating factor in triggering cancer. We also know that breaking the wall/barrier between a cancerous tumor and surrounding tissues as with biopsies, might aggravate or spread the disease. These tests and diagnostics are additionally known to give false positive results that can lead to more unnecessary testing and unwarranted treatments. Two of the worst side effects in cancer treatment, include suppression of the immune system, the most important healing system in the body, and a generalized inflammation which may in itself, cause more disease.

According to Western medicine, the possible mechanisms for spontaneous healing are theorized to be a combination of immune system function, psychological factors, spiritual influences and altered states of mind. To no surprise, these features fit right into the concept of expanding healing consciousness, gaining knowledge, understanding, having belief, faith and non-attachment to outcome, all triggering the body's biochemistry and immune system. In other words, they correlate with alignment of the five essential components for healing. The subject of spontaneous remission or healing would easily fill volumes of its own. It is important to understand that spontaneous healing is one of the possible results of aligning the five essential components for healing, bringing us to that place of knowingness that without a doubt, we will heal. And, spontaneous healing often takes place accidentally, without our realizing it, simply by the nature of innately aligning the five essential components for healing while having a powerful intention and desire to be well. Know that clinical data has been telling us for at least centuries how cancer is not an irreversible disease.

A simple example of unconscious or accidental healing of our self, might be that time when you were feeling all the symptoms of a bad cold coming on. Maybe having the body ache, a cough, sore throat, stuffy sinuses, light headed and feeling feverish. The symptoms you know *always* result in a cold, the ones laying you up for three days to a week. Every time you have had symptoms that badly, you always end up sick. But then there are also those times, when you have the first realization of cold symptoms and immediately said to yourself, "I refuse to get sick. I don't have time, I've got too much to do and under no circumstance will I get sick this time." In retrospect, you remember you did not get sick. There are times when this is all we need to not to get sick. To have that knowingness, the right frame of mind, the state of healing consciousness that aligns the five essential components for healing, triggering the body's autoimmune system to heal itself. While it may be difficult to understand right now, I know this to be true, whether we are dealing with a wound healing faster than would be expected or cancer that is not supposed to get better without a lot of aggressive treatment, yet, it somehow vanished on its own. In these cases, most people do not realize the significance of their role in actively triggering the healing process. Generally, we are so busy with life that we have little memory of the early symptoms of the cold/disease and how close we were to being ill, or the part we played in preventing or curing the disease. We just gratefully forget we were on the verge of illness. I'm sure you can think back to a time when you avoided getting sick even though it seemed inevitable. This resultant healing is not simply that you had some positive or happy thought chasing a potential illness away. The facts are, your highly focused thoughts, feelings and emotions, along with an underlying knowledge, understanding, belief and faith, without attachment to outcome, put order to your healing consciousness that aligned the five essential secrets for healing. This generated the physical and energetic nature of thoughts, that in-turn, stimulated the immune system, glands, tissues and organs in the body, altering your anatomy, physiology and biochemistry leading to the healing.

It is important to understand, that in the same manner we heal ourselves, the reverse is also true in that we can cause ourselves illness. In the examples noted above, we had the knowledge and understanding of what the cold symptoms could turn into, or what we were told about the way cancer symptoms would progress. We knew how we would feel when our body and mind was ailing from those conditions, the length of time it might take to get better or worse, while concurrently *knowing* exactly the way we would feel not being sick and instead, in perfect health. Then, rather than focusing and dwelling on the symptoms of illness that could only fill our minds and body with negative thoughts and behaviors that promote disease, we instead, innately tapped into that place of knowing how we feel in our state of perfect health and strength. What followed, was without conscious intention, without even realizing, we automatically visualized ourselves without the cold symptoms, without the illness or cancer and instead, stayed present to the moment focusing our attention on doing what we needed to be doing in our lives. Our healing consciousness aligned itself and the five essential components for healing, activating the autoimmune system to healing the body with little conscious awareness.

I referred to *visualization* of ourselves without symptoms of illness. This will be explained in more detail in chapter six, though in simple terms for those unfamiliar with the term, I am referring to seeing images with our mind's eye, of our body, tissues, organs and systems in a state of perfect health. This process may seem like a lot of work and be time intensive but, it can all take place in a matter of seconds, even a fraction of a second, almost without notice. It always comes back to the way we think, to the thoughts we have and our ability to achieve the knowingness that there is no other possibility outside of our being well and healthy. Consciously or unconsciously, we are doing this all the time with our own health and the well-being of others. Achieving this state of knowingness is often of greater importance than the treatment itself.

Homeostasis

My hope is that your awareness is expanding for the obvious nature of our mind and body to continuously heal itself. One of the primary ways the body maintains health is through an endless process of sustaining *homeostasis*. Homeostasis is a state of balance in the body. It is a biochemical and neuroanatomical balance that takes place in every cell, in all tissues and organs of the body. When this balance is not maintained illness develops. Most people who have some understanding of homeostasis, imagine the cells of the body or entire body itself, being in a happy state of balance for long periods of time, until some outside force (infection, cancer, disease) moves it off balance creating dysfunction or illness. As a result of this imbalance and dysfunction, those who think this way, assume that the body then releases hormones modifying biochemicals to reestablish balance and maintain health. But the reality is, homeostasis lasts only for the most minute fraction of a second, if even that. Our bodies are in-fact, constantly moving away from homeostasis, away from ideal function and towards illness. At the same time, the body undergoing and endless effort to re-balance itself. For an illustration in understanding how this process of homeostasis functions in balancing the body and creating health, I like to use an analogy of a commercial jet autopilot system. When we take-off on a commercial flight, let's say, from New York to Los Angeles, the pilot sets the autopilot flight system and we imagine that the plane moving on a straight, bee-line path, directly from one point to the other without variation. Even through turbulence and strong weather conditions that might jar the jet off course, it seems that the autopilot snaps the jet back onto the one-and-only, straight as an arrow heading. What happens instead, is that the jet is constantly going off course. It *never* just flies in a straight line. The job of the auto-flight system is to make continual adjustments, hundreds or even thousands of times every minute to keep the jet on the intended course. There is an endless quantity of actions taking place by the auto-flight system, including, modifying speed, velocity, altitude, left turn, right turn, left or right tilt, nose up, nose down, monitoring hydraulic pressure and hundreds of other calculations and modifications. The jet needs to follow the curve of the earth, otherwise we would end up in outer space. In the same manner, each cell of the body, each organ system and the body as-a-whole is continuously going off course, over functioning or under functioning. In other words, our body is endlessly moving towards a state of dysfunction or disease. Fortunately, at the same time, in every organ system and every cell, the body is working towards reestablishing homeostasis/balance. Homeostasis in the body differs from the jetliner's hundreds or thousands of changes that take place every minute. In the body, there are *hundreds of trillions* of biochemical reactions taking place *every second*. When we align the five essential components for healing, bringing our healing consciousness to that place of knowingness, the physical and energetic nature of our thoughts stimulate those same hormones and biochemicals that create homeostasis.

You might realize by now, the following:

a. How belief and faith alone are not enough to create permanent, swift healing, and why it is necessary to also have the foundation of knowledge and understanding, while exercising non-attachment to outcome.
b. Why no single treatment works one hundred percent of the time for all patients even with the same condition.
c. The way healing consciousness is reformatted in the process of aligning the five essential components for healing.
d. The reasons alignment of the five essential components for healing will determine the degree and permanence of healing.

Seeming miracles of healing can unfold when the five essential components for healing are aligned and we are brought to that place of knowingness. In chiropractic, they call those miracles, SCMs, short for a "Standard Chiropractic Miracles." What might be considered miraculous healings are quite common in all healthcare and healing practices, even if accidentally. One example of an SCM might be the common scenario where a patient comes in with extreme back pain. This pain may be so intense they are carried into the office. The patient might have severe back pain with a radiation of pain, numbness and/or tingling down a leg into the foot and include muscle weakness in their legs or feet. The doctor is completely focused and present to the patient in taking a thorough history, performing a comprehensive examination and explaining the condition to the patient in detail. She/he then designs a treatment plan, clearly describing the treatment and telling the patient how they are going to feel so much better following therapy. The doctor employs the prescribed treatments and answers any final questions by the patient. During this process, engrossed in purposeful communication with the patient and continuing clinical procedures, the blocks and barriers to healing are falling away. At the same time, the patient's healing consciousness is being reformatted to *know* they will heal from the prescribed treatment. In this process, they receive reassurance and comfort around any fears related to their condition, while thoughts and emotions of illness or injury are being refocused on the truth that they can and will heal. In combination, all these activities are bringing together alignment of the five essential components for healing. Once this is accomplished, the patient thoughts and feelings are advanced to that place of knowingness, allowing them to respond to treatment, exactly as they were told they would. That is when the magic happens, when the miracles of healing take place. The point of describing this process is to understand that the doctor or practitioner can create an opportunity to guide their patient/recipient towards aligning the essential components for healing and thereby moving them to that state of knowing they will heal.

Within every healthcare or healing practice, guiding someone to that place of knowingness occurs through very specific communication skills. Any time as a practitioner we are engaged with a patient or recipient for healing, intentionally or inadvertently, we are in fact altering their healing consciousness in some way. We want this modification of healing consciousness by the practitioner to be taking place in positive rather than negative ways. Communication by a practitioner if suppressive to a patient's state of healing consciousness through reinforcing fears and hopelessness, will fail to align the five essential components for healing. On the other hand, communication that is a positive and educational experience, from the perspective of guiding a patient toward hope and greater possibilities in healing or in curing their condition, will move them towards alignment of the essential components for healing. As an example, take a doctor giving a report of findings to a patient who has cancer. It is not uncommon in this situation, for a doctor approaching a patient to report something like, "Your cancer has a high mortality rate and if you don't have radiation and chemotherapy right away, you will die in a few weeks. And, there is no guarantee even with all the treatment that you will survive for very long." This type of statement only creates fear and lack of hope, leaving no room for knowing anything other than an inevitability of becoming very sick and probably dying soon. On the other hand, a doctor who makes a statement to the patient such as, "While your cancer is quite advanced, there is really no telling how it might respond to treatment in your case. There have been cases where this cancer has gone into remission for many years, even patients living out their full productive life. While the medical model for this type of cancer is to prescribe chemotherapy and radiation (explaining the potential benefits and disadvantages), there are additional and alternative options for treating the cancer that you can incorporate at the same time. It is important to use tools that boost your mental and emotional health, support your immune system and be as physically active as is possible." The doctor additionally gives the patient resources and guidance to manage their health and treatment. In this second case, the doctor is guiding the patient towards altering their state of healing consciousness, allowing alignment of the five essential components for healing, triggering healthful, restorative thoughts that translate to healing changes in the body.

One of our goals as a physician or healing practitioner is to avoid unintentionally enabling a patient's state of healing consciousness to remain stuck in old, limiting patterns of thinking and belief related illness and healing. This would only move their state of mind towards preventing healing or worsening a condition. In the same manner, when we are facing our own health issues, we want to practice expanding our perspective on how illness and healing take place, broadening our healing consciousness to better guide our body in the direction of health. Know that the doctor or practitioner is only one part of the equation for healing, it takes more than going to a doctor to be well. The doctor and practitioner are the principle guides in the process of managing illness. They are one of the tools we utilize in doing everything we can to align the five essential components for healing. Ultimately, and in conjunction with all medical and alternative care, healing from any illness whether we are addressing the sniffles or cancer, always comes back to the way we are thinking. In other words, the degree and permanence of healing depends on our own thoughts, feelings and emotions.

As a medical or alternative healing practitioner, it is important to understand that the process of altering a patient/recipient's healing consciousness begins from the first moment they enter the office door. This includes, the type of greeting and attention they receive from the staff and the initial introduction to the practitioner. There is an immediate energetic connection or repulsion between the practitioner and patient. However, it unfolds, this relationship will almost immediately affect all possibilities for healing, creating or preventing limitations to healing and affecting the potential response to care. By this, I mean, if the patient feels supported and cared for by the office and have a positive relationship with the doctor, their healing consciousness is already being elevated, setting up a greater chance of a beneficial response to treatment. On the other hand, if a patient feels uncomfortable or apprehensive about the office and fails to feel a trustful connection with the doctor, these patients will be protective of their limiting beliefs around illness and healing, preventing guidance toward expanding their healing consciousness and aligning the essential components for healing. Their chances for a positive response to treatment will then be reduced.

People develop a very deep attachment to the unique way they understand their illness and how they *believe* healing is going to take place or not. This understanding and belief may be misaligned with the reality of their condition. Prior to seeing a doctor, most people now days have likely discussed their condition with family or friends and at least researched it through the Internet. In this process, they are filled with more information, possibly adding new fixed ideas about their condition that may not be accurate or true. This being the case, the patient arrives to the practitioner's office with their own ideas of what ailment they have and how it should be treated. Once in the treatment room, the average practitioner having learned a specific and often narrow set of procedures and protocols for figuring out what a problem is, performs some type of history and examination or assessment on the patient. Following that history and exam, the doctor arrives at a diagnosis utilizing their knowledge, references for differentiating disease in their specialty or refer to the latest textbooks. They have additional references for prescribing medication, treatment and therapies depending on the specific diagnosis. A practitioner's knowledge may be keen, intuitive, holistic and up-to-date. On other hand, a doctor may be practicing in the same way they always have, not taking a patient's uniqueness into account and following their own fixed, limiting references and protocols. A physician or healing practitioner needs to have an awareness that patients/recipients arrive with preconceived ideas about their condition. This allows them to explore their perspective on illness, their expectations regarding treatment and find ways to guide the patient toward broadening their healing consciousness and greater possibilities for healing. In addition to the patient's healing consciousness, we want to realize that the practitioner has his or her own underlying state of healing consciousness. A doctor's perspective on illness and healing may also be broad and expansive or filled with their own fixed prejudices for healing. Expectations of both the practitioner and patient are best aligned to create trust and the knowingness they will heal. The bottom line is, communication and the relationship developed between the practitioner and patient is important in expanding healing consciousness and aligning the five essential components for healing.

My intention is that we increase our ability to deliberately and purposefully align the five essential components for healing, triggering the body's natural ability to repair itself. In chapter six, I share tools for broadening healing consciousness and enhancing our ability to purposefully and intentionally bring ourselves to that place of knowingness.

Present-Time Communication and Aligning The Five Secret Components for Healing Yourself and Others

Part of the process of aligning the five essential components for healing, requires *trusting the practitioner*. The greater the trust in the practitioner, the better the response to treatment. In order to develop a belief and faith in the healing process, the patient needs to trust that the knowledge and understanding they are gaining from the practitioner is true. This knowledge and understanding about the patient's condition as presented by the practitioner needs to be clear and accurate. Initial communication between the practitioner and patient will be a key element in building a foundation of belief and faith for healing. From the development of knowledge, understanding, belief and faith, also comes the basis for establishing trust. This trust in the doctor can be a large part of generating the knowingness that you are capable of healing, thereby allowing non-attachment to outcome, the fifth essential component for healing. The result can be the definitive knowingness, that without a doubt, healing will take place. If trust in the practitioner is absent or incomplete, the five essential components for healing will be out of alignment. Think about the times when the most exact and appropriate treatment is prescribed or performed, and it fails to help the condition in the slightest degree. This can be true even for an antibiotic. How many times are antibiotics taken for a widespread infection where some people respond, and others do not? There might be a time when a patient is sitting across the desk from their physician who is prescribing that antibiotic, where the patient might be thinking, "Well, I don't have an infection, it is just sinus inflammation and an antibiotic is going to do nothing." The result being, based on that patient's healing consciousness, they lack the knowledge, belief or trust in the doctor. As a result, they may fail to respond to the prescribed treatment or even improve before they begin the antibiotic. Knowing that thoughts change biochemistry, this patient feeling/knowing deep within their being that they have no infection, in that moment, their immune system is instantly set in motion eradicating any infection. While to some this may seem phenomenal, it is in-fact, a common result of the powerful energy of our thoughts triggering biochemical changes in the body.

Following is an example of how important being completely present to the patient or recipient, instills knowledge, understanding, belief, faith and trust in their healing process. As previously noted, this takes place through highly focused communication, reformatting their healing consciousness and thereby aligning the five essential components for healing. This example will be from my chiropractic orthopedic perspective. While reading the following example, relate this illustration to your own type of practice as this model easily applies to every type of physician or healing practitioner. In all communication with patients, the first key is being completely present to the patient, them with you and without inner or outer distractions. There is no thinking about the past or the future. You want to be completely present with all your heart and soul, to every patient.

Here are two examples to make this point;

Patient #1

> A new patient comes into the office and they are sitting across from you at your desk. You are completely and totally present to them. You are not thinking about the last patient or the next. You are not being distracted by a recent phone call and your staff has instructions to avoid interrupting you during a consultation. There is nothing

on your mind or in your thoughts, other being present, focused and caring for this important human being who seeks your guidance and assistance for their health issue. You take them through a thorough and focused history of the patient's past and current health condition, especially probing for activities, behaviors, emotional issues and lifestyle concerns that may have contributed to their complaint or condition (What is important here is understanding the thoroughness and presence to the patient, rather than why or what questions are being asked.). You listen to every word from a perspective of compassion, understanding, and holistic analysis. Then, bringing them into the examination room, you perform a comprehensive global and local examination to rule-out some conditions and to specifically define the problem. You can always tell when a patient present and absorbed in the process, listening to every word you say, thoroughly engaged and watching every movement you make. Their eyes are tracking your every move, they respond to each instruction you give, and nothing distracts them. You know they are completely connected to you and absorbed in your process of assessment. The patient is in a place of trust, knowing that their best interest is your most important concern in that moment. Arriving at a diagnosis, you clearly explain their condition to them using models, charts, book images or computer graphics. I kept a library in my primary treatment room of books and references with literally every possible condition tabbed for quick access. I could easily show patients images of how their condition appeared in its current state of ill-health, on a large scale or cellular level. Meaning, pictures of the way an entire organ appeared, maybe a lung or kidney with lesions and how the damaged tissue cells appear within those organs. Whether disease involved bone, muscle, nerve, tendon, cartilage, circulation, kidneys, lungs or any other tissue, this would give the patient knowledge and understanding of their present state. In doing this, the patient would have visual images in their minds of how their diseased or damaged tissues might appear as a reference point, then also present illustrations of the same tissues in their normal and healthy state. This is part of broaden a patient's healing consciousness and aligning the five essential components for healing. Giving them clear visual references for both how their tissues appear in the current state of dysfunction and in perfect health, I am able guide the energy of their thoughts and feelings, in other words, guide their minds eye toward seeing those tissues move from a place of disease, to their most healthy state.

I would then design a treatment plan, explain to the patient in detail what the treatment consisted of, how it would be employed, the intended effects on the damaged tissues (as in the images I presented to them), how those tissues would respond and return to their normal healthy state. The patient would receive reassurance that it was possible for them to heal and told how great they would be feeling after the treatment and in the days to follow. This conversation was all geared toward reformatting their healing consciousness and aligning the essential components. Treatment might have included any of the following, myofascial release work, an adjustment, stretching of the tissues and physiotherapy modalities such as, ultrasound, muscle stimulation, motorized traction, hot, cold or electrical modalities. In my experience, this type of meticulous patient management, modifies healing consciousness, altering the body's biochemical and neurochemical functions trigger healing, and will be at least as important if not much more than the treatment applied. Lastly, the patient would be prescribed some type of home care treatment to promote thoughts and actions that support the continued healing. These might include any combination of stretches, exercises, ergonomic recommendations for work, home or sleep, nutritional guidance or emotional support. Maintaining complete presence to the patient throughout this process is essential.

Almost every time a patient is treated in this manner, they would leave the office feeling just as I said they would, better or improved. These patients would go home telling all their family and friends about the wonderful care they received. They are happy people who continually fill your practice with more happy patients. This form of healing takes place when we are unconditionally present and connected with our patient/client. Their healing consciousness is broadened, they align the five essential components for healing in that process and are brought to that place of knowingness, where without a doubt, they will heal. This is when the magic of healing takes place for literally every condition. It is when the magic of healing takes place in every healthcare or healing office. Just to be clear, when I'm talking about the miracle of healing, rather than meaning a religious experience of sorts, with angels from heaven touching us with healing, I am referring to the miracle that healing is every time it takes place and the miracle of our body's innate ability to affect its own healing process. The miracle is the way nature creates vitality and balance to the world in every aspect, including healing disease.

Patient #2

Then, in a contrasting example, you have another new patient, only this time you are distracted and not completely present. Maybe you are just running behind with patients, hungry with low blood sugar, having problems with staff in the office, having your own physical pain or thinking about relationship problems at home. You might be dealing with issues surrounding your children, thinking about an upcoming vacation, having financial worries or thinking about other work you need to be doing. This new patient sits across the desk from you and begins to tell you what is bothering them. Within the first ninety seconds of taking this history, you realize all they need is an adjustment of the fifth lumbar vertebrae and sacral joints (L5/S1) at the bottom of the spine and they'll be feeling great. That being clear and now fixed in your mind, you cut taking the history and move them into the exam room. A simple cursory examination seems to be in order because you have already decided that once L5/S1 are adjusted, the patient's back will be completely fine. The truth is, in chiropractic, all 365 bones in the body including fingers, toes, ears and nose, can be adjusted in less than three minutes. Generally, this type of quick adjustment spanning every joint in the body, will fail to create the trust or expansion of healing consciousness necessary for the patient to achieve that state of knowing they will heal, especially a first-time patient. I will point out though, there are patients who love and respond perfectly well to this type of quick adjustment. Some will come into the office and say something like, "I've only got five minutes for a quick adjustment." These patients do respond perfectly to that style of treatment, though it is more typical for longtime patients experiencing a flare-up for a known condition or seeking preventative care. These patients have previously been through and experienced the consultation/examination, where they gained the knowledge, understanding, trust and expanded healing consciousness that allows alignment of the five essential components for healing. They already know the great value and benefits of an adjustment and have that knowingness they will feel better after treatment. But in my experience, this is not the case for most patients, especially new patients who are yet to have the knowledge, understanding, belief, faith and non-attachment to out-come necessary to align the five essential components for healing.

In these cases where you have predetermined that all the patient needed was an adjustment, you might only perform a cursory examination and quickly offer the patient a minimal explanation of their condition and needs. Rather than defining an accurate and specific diagnosis, you might tell them something general, such as, "you strained your back," or give a simple, commonly heard but incorrect diagnosis like, "you have a pinched nerve." A "pinched nerve" diagnosis is most often, a way the practitioner avoids spending time explaining the details of a patient's condition. The next step in this example, you tell the patient you are going to give them an adjustment. You offer no clear description of their condition, haven't described the exact nature of treatment, nor have you related the way their body might respond. The adjustment you provide to them, though, is the most perfect adjustment for their body type and condition. One of those great magical adjustments, the one that would part the Red Sea. The adjustment that would clear the clouds from the heavens and warm the earth with love and light. It all happens very quickly, and you tell the patient, "great, see you next time." The problem is, the adjustment didn't help. The patient stands up from the table feeling no better and maybe even worse. Even though they are not satisfied with the visit, they are rushed out of the treatment room to make a follow-up appointment and were unable to tell you how they were feeling.

This patient most often leaves the office very unhappy. They are not feeling better, may be feeling worse and at least subconsciously, feeling uncared for. They might go home, tell their family and friends that the treatment was useless and may not return for their follow-up visit. But no, these patients always return. Only at their next appointment, not only is their condition no better, but they have all sorts of additional complaints. Instead of just having the original lower back pain, they now have pain on the right side of their neck, a headache, their left shoulder hurts and all sorts of new ailments have arisen. Most often these new complaints make no clinical sense based on their condition and the treatment applied, though they all need to be addressed. With these new complaints, you are now forced into spending the time being present to this patient, in the way you could have been during the initial visit. Being completely present, you now explain in detail what their condition is, how they got that way, what exactly their diagnosis means, what the treatment consists of, why they failed to respond to the initial treatment and how exactly the treatment will make a difference in their condition. In other words, spending the time being present, expanding their healing consciousness, aligning the essential components for healing, with knowledge, understanding and trust that you could have created at the initial visit.

In this second example, one or more of the five essential components for healing were out of alignment. The patient was clearly lacking knowledge, understanding, belief, faith and non-attachment to outcome required to bring them to that place of knowing they would heal. They lacked trust in the practitioner. The first example in comparison, the practitioner was completely present to the patient, the five essential components for healing were aligned and the patients healing consciousness was guided to the place of knowing they would heal. Where in the second example, a perfect treatment was rendered with a poor outcome, a successful response in the first example would have taken place even applying a mediocre or adequate treatment.

The necessity of being completely present in the process of aligning the five essential components for healing is the same no matter what type of healthcare or healing practice you have. The effects of being present to the patient, instilling appropriate knowledge and understanding, creating belief and faith, will bring them to that state of knowingness they will heal. While this was an example in a chiropractic practice, the same will be true for any form of medicine or healing. From the moment the patient/recipient enters your office, makes initial contact with you the practitioner, the degree and permanence of healing will depend on your being completely present to them. In this way, you can guide them away from limiting thoughts related to illness and health, reformatting their healing consciousness and allowing alignment of the five essential components for healing.

I cannot emphasize enough, the importance of having total presence to your patient/recipient. In all my years of clinical practice, it would be difficult for me to tell you the number of times a patient returned feeling so much better or healed, that I wondered if they had improved from the hands-on, manual treatment and all the machines, or if they had gotten better through our relationship and healing guidance. It seemed their healing evolved to a greater degree, through the process of reformatting of their healing consciousness and aligning the five essential components for healing, before, during and after the treatment.

This process of bringing a patient to that place of knowingness, within the deepest fabric of their being that they will heal, can be more important than the treatment itself. When the recipient achieves that state of knowingness, they will respond to most any form of treatment whether through the intervention of medication, radiation, surgery, hands-on manual therapy or energy therapies. This is when the energy of our thoughts and feelings become most concentrated and focused, stimulating the biochemical process in the body that jump starts the immune system and healing. In other words, this is when the physical and energetic nature of the energy of our thoughts, trigger glands, tissues and organs to release specific chemicals in the body that regulate healing. Whether we are dealing with something as simple as a cut on a finger, an antibiotic for an infection, surgery or chemotherapy and radiation for cancer, the effect is the same. When the five essential components for healing are aligned, even a placebo will stimulate the body's healing process.

*"We are what we think. All that we are arises with our
thoughts. With our thoughts, we make the world."*

GAUTAMA BUDDHA

Reaching that state of knowingness always comes back to the
way we are thinking. From thoughts we have on a daily-basis to
thoughts related to how we understand illness and healing. Every
thought and feeling we have, positive or negative, will affect the
way we heal. We experience 60,000 to 80,000 thoughts a day, each
one having a profound effect on our general and specific state of
health, right down to our genetic coding. Each thought we have is
impacting our anatomy and physiology making positive or negative
changes. Consciously or unconsciously, every thought is flipping
switches in the body, stimulating glands that secrete hormones,
triggering chemicals that are productive and regenerative or
destructive, altering our anatomy and physiology on a cellular level.
While the subject of another book I'm currently working on, the
simplest way to describe this affect is through the latest research
on what scientists have termed *The Placebome Effect*. In the
Placebome effect, researchers compared patients in a study taking
placebos who responded in the same manner or better as patients
taking the true medication. These placebo patients showed identical neurochemical reactions in the brain, triggering the same biochemical response in the body as those taking the medicine. They
also found that the patients taking the placebo showed identical,
permanent alteration of their DNA as those taking the medication.
This is a remarkable finding, proving that the effects of a placebo
are not just in the mind, but have true anatomical and physiological
effects. It also confirms the fact, that every thought, feeling and
emotion we have, carries the capability of moving our body in the
direction of illness or health. Our thoughts can cause or reduce

inflammation in the body, elevate or depress our mood, build or damage cells, give us energy or shut down the mind and body, make us feel anxious, depressed and sad or lift our spirits to blissful joy. It always comes back to the way we are thinking. The more we understand the nature of thoughts and emotions, as physical and energetic entities, the greater we will understand our ability to guide the energy of those thoughts in healing ourselves and others.

Know that when I'm speaking about of the healing energy of thoughts, I'm not talking about *positive thinking*, where we might have happy thoughts that make us feel better in some way, thereby reducing an amount of discomfort. This may distract us from our illness and maybe help us "feel" better or improved from something that is not a serious health issue. When I refer to the energy of a thought, I am specifically talking about the scientifically defined nature of a thought as both a *physical particle* and a *wave of energy*. In my practice of BioCognitive Healing, we guide those physical and energetic properties of *thought energy* to stimulate specific glands, tissues, systems and organs, in triggering the body's innate healing response and capabilities.

"If you carry joy in your heart, you can heal any moment."

CARLOS SANTANA

Why Some People Fail to Heal, Obstacles and Barriers to Knowingness

While this can be an uncomfortable subject, let us look at some of the more conscious and self-generated reasons for why some people *may not want to heal.*

Any one of us might, at separate times in our lives and for different conditions based on our state of healing consciousness, our life experience related to healing up to the point of an illness in our lives, might consciously or unconsciously choose not to heal. According to behavioral scientists, countless psychological, psychosocial, psychobiological and personal reasons exist for not wanting to heal. A vast majority of those reasons are unconscious. Freud called this type of illness or lack of healing, the result of *primary* and *secondary gains.* The primary gains from illness would be the creation of thoughts and behaviors that generate positive internal feelings about oneself. This patient might feel good about going to the best doctors and facilities or having some time for rest and relaxation. Secondary gains from illness are what he describes as *extorting proofs*, meaning we manipulate someone else in order to have them take care of us, or do things for us that prove their love. In other words, extorting love or support for our beliefs about illness from another person. A secondary gain could also be defined, as an excuse to explain or avoid having not made the effort or taken a risk to be successful in a task or profession where we feel we *should* have been. A secondary gain can be a used as proof that we are not able to accomplish something we thought we could and wanted to achieve. Any manner of not wanting to heal for most people is highly unconscious, presenting as a deeply rooted pattern of thinking or behavior. Unfortunately, we are not likely to even be aware or know if we are sabotaging our healing, because it's unconscious! And those who might get a glimpse of their part in not healing or even those who know they are choosing not to heal, would unlikely be willing or may be unable to acknowledge to others that they are not wanting to be better. In a situation where someone has the awareness of not wanting to get better, would most likely feel shameful or embarrassed, especially feeling as if they were lacking the tools to be able to change those thoughts and feelings. Because of their present state of healing consciousness, they might feel completely powerless and incapable of thinking or acting in any other fashion. This can bring great frustration, maybe depression and reinforce an ongoing illness.

Unconscious reasons for not wanting to improve or heal can be simple or highly complex. Either way, when you are in the middle of these unconscious limiting thoughts and feeling patterns around illness, it is not so easy to identify or reverse them. In psychobiological and psychosocial terms, it might be said that there is a *payoff* of sorts for staying ill. Noted psychologist Eric Berne in his book, "The Games People Play," refers to these secondary gains as "benefits of illness." He says that in these situations, staying in a place of illness is less painful than confronting a life challenge that appears insurmountable. The suffering is not great enough to move someone in making life changes that would promote healing. Berne says that people even seek surgeries in the face of medical opposition to avoid some part of life's responsibilities, or possibly a way to receive the related attention from doctors, hospital staff and probably more important, from partners, family or friends.

While illness-payoffs may occur to varying degrees in anyone facing illness, it is of course not always the case, nor the only reason for not healing. We are all unique in our state of healing consciousness. Even the most consciously evolved person, may exhibit the proper perspective in aligning the five essential components for healing related to one type of health issue, but not for another. And commonly, when someone is not using an illness for primary or secondary gain, they are more likely to be avoiding the attention surrounding healthcare or at times, even being in denial about the need to see a doctor. While the following list may seem coarse to some, others will find these illustrations as a reality check or obvious examples. Be open to the possibility that these types of issues could be involved with the way you and others heal or not.

Reasons some people may fail to heal:

1. To avoid dealing with a difficult situation. These might include difficulties in relationships, a hardship in business, issues with children, work, family, school, career or in financial crises.
2. As a way of getting attention, feeling loved or proof of being loved and cared for.
3. As a reason to avoid responsibilities, such as, going to work or school, avoid participating in household chores and duties.
4. Avoidance of conflict, at home, in relationships, at work or with friends.
5. As an attempt to avoid connecting with a spouse, partner, family member or friend.
6. Rather than confront and deal with feelings of low self-esteem, failure or feelings of unworthiness, staying in a place of ill-health as with depression, loneliness and indecision.
7. In order to *feel* something in one's life. To feel anything, even pain, rather than being numbed out to life and feeling nothing.

8. A reason to be intolerant, have destructive behaviors, rage or to be left alone.
9. To gain sympathy, compassion or empathy.
10. There might be monetary compensation for a disability as with an automobile accident, lawsuit or work injury.
11. A reason or excuse for not having achieved something, gained a material goal or reached a certain desired level of life success.
12. An excuse for not having a relationship, not taking the risk of putting oneself out in the single's world, or to justify a feeling of loneliness and lack of love.
13. Being in a state of illness avoids facing some of fears, making it difficult or impossible to take healthy, appropriate risks in one's life.
14. Generally, a defensive mechanism for not participating in life. A reason for being lazy.
15. Illness can create the feeling of a *lack of meaning or purpose* in life, reducing the desire of trying to be better or creating a life purpose.
16. In reverse of number 15, some people find meaning and purpose in their illness. They are consumed with dealing in their medical problems, consumed with being in all the right places for their care and leaving no room to be doing anything else. This one can take you back to the top of the list in a cycle of reasons to be ill or not get well.

As an example, think about a person who might be going through a very difficult and challenging relationship at home or work. A relationship where they have long felt unloved, unappreciated, with low self-esteem and feelings of unworthiness. They are unable to express how they have been feeling, possibly been physically or emotionally abused, run a household and care for children, never getting a break, continually exhausted and functioning from a place of resentment and frustration. Becoming ill for someone in this situation might create many secondary gains. They would have the opportunity for feeling forced into taking a break due to illness, thereby creating time to rest and recover from what is, rather than illness, a really an uncomfortable and out-of-control feeling about their life. This results in attention and care from family, friends and healthcare providers. They receive sympathy and help from family and friends, thereby feeling loved, as well as a reduction of responsibilities at work and home that were causing them stress. When this person is sick or dealing with illness, they don't have time to dealing with the usual daily stresses, and instead can refocus their attention on a hamster wheel of doctor's appointments and medical tests. These findings corroborate with an abundance of evidence over many decades, confirming our ability to cause ourselves serious illness by the way we think and feel.

Another inner experience that can cause depression and disease, are feelings of unworthiness or low self-esteem. Even without life situations of external physical or emotional abuse from relationships or work, even in the face of great life success, anyone might at some time in their lives experience feelings of low self-esteem for not having achieved their own unique and specific desired life goals. Feelings of failure can arise for not having the dream relationship they desired, for not having things they thought they wanted, the right amount of money, children or the ideal place to live. Feelings of unworthiness and low-self-esteem can also be the basis for illness that brings about secondary gains. Secondary incentives might include fear of spending time or taking the necessary risks on tasks that could bring a desired life success. "I'm feeling too depressed or unworthy to put myself out or take those actions." These feelings might create a sense of hopelessness, an incapacity to pursue a relationship and avoid risks of failure or embarrassment in relationships and business. Secondary gains can simply be excuses. These types of life stresses often bring compassionate supporters and enablers who validate the problems, while not helping to create a solution.

The above list and examples are not presented to make anyone feel bad or incapable of healing themselves. They are not meant to infer that emotional and psychosocial secondary gains are always the only reasons for creating illness, or that we should always be able to simply heal ourselves and others. Emotional components of illness and thoughts interfering with healing are deeply subconscious issues, rooted in our healing consciousness from an early age. Reformatting healing consciousness to greater possibilities, takes highly intentional work. If your life perspective is one of *total accountability*, meaning that you take full responsibility for creating everything that takes place in your life, every life situation, every person and event that takes place in your life, you will already have an easier grasp of this subject. But that is not the case for most people. Most people require a significant amount of guidance, training and support to effectively remove the mind's blocks and barriers in expand their healing consciousness. This is what I have been practicing and teaching for more than forty years as a healthcare provider and now in the practice Bio-Cognitive Healing.

The process of expanding our healing consciousness and aligning the five essential components for healing, as is true for anything else, might be natural to some people, while taking more work and practice for others. It is important to understand that our healing consciousness is constantly evolving. Whatever our skills in healthcare and healing might be in this moment, whether as a seasoned practitioner or being all together new to this growing sphere of healing, there will always be room for continued improvement of our ability and skills in healing ourselves and others.

A question I'm often asked at retreats is this, "If it just takes believing in the physician, having knowledge, understanding and believing the therapy is going to work, why am I not getting better? I was believing, trusting my doctor, even saying daily affirmations that I am in perfect health and healing in the best way possible. So why am I not healed?" The first part of an answer to this question is that it can be easy to sincerely say the words, "I am believing." But the problem with having this thought is that even with the best of intentions, regularly meditating, routinely saying affirmations and visualizing improvement, the reality of healing thoughts, are far more complex than simply *saying*, I believe.

The truth of authentic belief or more specifically, reaching that place of *knowingness*, takes place beyond unconscious, automatic thought and expression, beyond our ability to logically and intentionally desire or deliberately state that we believe. Sometimes people are "trying so hard" to believe they can be better, while those thoughts are being counter acted upon by so many deeply ingrained, subconscious layers of learned limitations and barriers around illness. Most people hold so tightly to their mental blocks and obstacles around healing, that even with the sincerest intentional desires of *trying* to believe, will more often result in great amounts of *wishing and hoping*. Wishing and hoping does not carry the same effects on our body as than having the knowingness that they will be better. There are so many possibilities surrounding illness and health, from progressively getting worse, having no change, gaining slight improvement, going into remission, having partial healing, full healing or being completely cured. What I have learned and practiced over many decades is that the progression of either healing or worsening will depend to the greatest degree, on our current state of healing consciousness. While our healing consciousness is inherently filled with obstacles and barriers to healing that we have carried throughout our lives, there is good news. We have the capability of reformatting our healing consciousness by altering the way we understand illness and through modifying or removing those mental barriers to healing. We can then better cultivate our healing conscious in ways that intentionally improve our skills at aligning the five essential components for healing, bringing ourselves and others to that place of knowing we will heal.

Our subconscious mind, though, so frequently and organically, sabotages our desire to heal. Our nature is to hold firmly to old ideas related healing, even the ones that may not be true. Even though we might work diligently at being highly conscious in all areas of our lives, including around health, preconceived thoughts, beliefs and barriers to healing, are embedded in the deepest recesses of our mind. They are subconscious. Having no conscious awareness of those thoughts and behaviors that are automatically governed by the unconscious mind, it is difficult to reformat those blocks and barriers on our own. So how do we change them?

We now understand that most limiting thoughts and obstacles to healing are acquired during our early years of being raised. This takes place when our healing consciousness is forming, especially during the period between birth and about age eight. These limitations can seriously inhibit our ability not only to heal, but also constrain our capability for manifesting so many other desires, such as, relationships, careers and valuable life goals. We are born into this world, as pure, unadulterated, capable healers with innate abilities in manifesting health. The problem is that as newborns and infants, we are without the physical ability to communicate our knowledge or even fully understand those abilities in relation to the new world around us. Prior to learning all the reason healing cannot take place, from spiritual and mystical points of view, many people including myself, believe babies and infants heal themselves and their families all the time. We know through science that babies and children heal faster than adults. Whether cuts, broken bones, cancer or responding to treatments for most every illness, babies are faster at healing. Let us now look even deeper into the way that these mental blocks and barriers to healing are formed.

The Brain
Location and Processing, of Thoughts and Memories that Form Blocks and Barriers to Healing

To better understand limitations to healing, we want to look at how these blocks and barriers are formed and etched into our healing consciousness. In our sensitive and vulnerable years from birth to age eight, we are inundated with other people's behaviors, actions, patterns of thinking and beliefs, not all of which will serve us well. We are influenced by every person we encounter. Throughout these times, we are forming permanent life perspectives, beliefs and turning them into indelible memories that we will live by. Through observation, the simple act of watching our role models, sometimes consciously other times unconsciously at the periphery of our awareness, we listen to what they say, observe their actions and behaviors, witness the way they function, including their reactions to illness and health. Some people internalize all this information, becoming so rigorously attached to what they learn and observe from their caregivers, they may go their entire existence as if living someone else's life. In other words, they go their entire lives behaving and thinking, exactly as a parent or caregiver who raised them in every respect. They never become their own unique selves, with their own mindful, creative thoughts, actions and behaviors. Living one's life in this fashion would be almost completely unconscious and unintentional, deeply rooted in the mind and spirit. This might be true in the ways we think and behave in relationships, in our career, related to our health, religion, in raising our children, in the ways we behave, react and respond to others. You might think of it as being a clone of a parent or caregiver. Renowned poet and playwright, Oscar Wilde, who we know as an avid non-conformist and creative thinker, was quoted as saying "Most people are other people. Their thoughts are someone else's opinions, their lives a mimicry, their passions a quotation." Ideally through our lives, we grow into our unique selves, having our own minds, thoughts and behaviors. We mature into being able to make our own distinct life choices, express our individual selves, have our own behaviors and reactions, while evolving into more conscious and conscientious people. Rather than be stuck with outdated, learned thinking around health, this book is focused on guiding the development of our own unique perspective on illness and healing. In other words, reformatting our healing consciousness through stripping away old layers of limiting information, removing blocks and barriers to healing, while at the same time, letting it be okay for healing to take place in ways we never thought possible.

In these early years when our healing consciousness is developed, most all the information we absorb, constructs a very narrow and tightly knit perspective of what we will understand and believe about illness, medical care and the way we are supposed to heal. This is not a judgement on how we were raised. We are all reared based on the best knowledge our parents have at that time, based on what they learned and perceived about illness and health, supplemented by our own developing perspective and interpretation. However, our growing minds process and store the information around health, it will be our healing consciousness that determines the degree we are able to align the five essential components for healing and achieve the state of know we will heal ourselves and others.

Earlier in the book I gave an example of a skewed perspective on health, whereby as children, our parents would call the doctor anytime someone was sick. This would result in the idea that, "If you don't go to the doctor when you are sick, you won't get better." We know people go to the doctor all the time with illness and disease that even where the most appropriate treatment prescribed, not everyone is improved or cured. Sometimes people are properly diagnosed, treated and respond to treatment and while others are not. There are times when conditions are not accurately diagnosed, fail to be treated properly and are not cured. We find that not only does medicine have its limitations, but that human beings are so unique in every way, including how they are injured and heal, even with what might *appear* to be the same injury or illness. This is well illustrated when studying human anatomy through dissection. In the laboratory, no two cadaver's joints are shaped exactly alike. Nerves appear in different anatomical locations from one body to another and when compared to images in the medical books. Most all tissues of the body present themselves in a variety of sizes, shapes, location and positions than how they appear in any anatomy dissection text. This reminds us that with an unlimited variation in uniqueness of anatomy and differences in physiology, along with each individual's unique state of healing consciousness, that even with the same diagnosis, very few people will respond to treatment in the *exact* same manner. In addition, not all doctors are created equally. As with any other profession, there highly skilled, conscientious practitioners, some with a natural ability for their healing art and other doctors who practice on autopilot, by-the-book, without being sensitive to each patient's unique history and relationship with illness and health. In all illness and healing, it always comes back to the ways we are thinking, the state of our healing consciousness and ability to modify old knowledge, understanding and beliefs. To better understand some of the reasons for our healing or not, I am going to describe the locations in the brain where these blocks and barriers are processed and stored.

Creation, Processing and Storage, of Limiting Thoughts, Blocks and Barriers to Healing in the Brain.

I'm going to describe two specific regions of the brain that administrate, coordinate and permanently fix memories. This is where our thoughts and behaviors are etched within the brain's neuroanatomy, and on an even deeper level, within our spiritual selves. These areas are involved with our automatic unconscious behaviors. From these locations in the brain, emerge involuntary expressions of our knowledge, judgements, our understanding, beliefs and faith on every subject, including illness and healing. They are also the locations where mental obstacles, and limitations to healing are processed and potentially set in stone. It is where our healing consciousness is developed and enduringly fixed. Understanding this process will allow us greater access and awareness in reformatting healing consciousness, by removing and modifying blocks to healing ourselves and others.

The Prefrontal Cortex

The first area of the brain I will address is the *prefrontal cortex*, sometimes called "the most human part of the brain," due to it being larger and more developed in humans compared to any other mammal. This is the area where we store and process *explicit memory*, also referred to as *declarative memory*. Located anatomically at the front of the brain, the prefrontal cortex is the region of *executive function*, orchestrating our cognitive thoughts, behaviors and the way we express ourselves. This activity being located anatomically at the front of our brain is similarly at the forefront of our thinking or conscious mind. This being the case, as important as the prefrontal cortex is in everyday function, it surprisingly makes up only about 10% of our thoughts, actions and how we express ourselves. This is where our *conscious thinking* resides, where explicit memory is processed and coordinated. The prefrontal cortex might be considered the logical, intellectual and analytical area of the brain. It is where we consciously and intentionally process information, have reasoning and problem-solving skills. From the prefrontal cortex, we determine right from wrong, orchestrate intentions, experience creative thoughts and ideas, make decisions, store and express facts and have vocabulary. From this part of the brain, we can carry on conversations about food, science, news and politics. It is from the prefrontal cortex that our inventive mind conceives and creates new life objectives, the location of expressing our personalities, and from where we might describe as what is fundamentally, ourselves. Having control of the pre-frontal cortex is not fully developed until our twenties, reducing a person's ability to exercise self-control until they have matured.

The Amygdala / The Old Brain

The second location in the brain related to processing and utilizing thoughts and behavior highly important to healing consciousness is the *Amygdala*, also called *the Old Brain*. The amygdala is located on each side at the base of the brain and is only about the side of an almond. This is where another type of memory is processed and expressed, *Implicit Memory* or *Procedural Memory*. Activity in the amygdala makes up a whopping 90% of our thoughts, behaviors, actions and self-expressions. The Old Brain is activated spontaneously from earlier acquired ideas, thoughts and beliefs, based on well-learned previous experience and practice. You might think about this area in relation to the *unconscious* mind. One example of procedural memory might be related to being potty trained as child. Initially, it is the prefrontal cortex working to figure out and understand the meaning and process of exercising control in using a bathroom. With time and repetition, the process becomes etched into the *amygdala* and no longer relies on the prefrontal cortex or conscious mind to monitor potty control. It becomes automatic. This is a process of writing the practice of control into the *subconscious mind*. Also referred to as procedural memory, this is the area of the brain giving us the capability for performing tasks on autopilot without having to place all our attention on every detail of a task. For instance, we use our implicit or procedural memory when riding a bicycle or driving a car. In these situations, we might be able to think about other things or carry on a conversation while not paying full focused attention on every detail of a task. As an example, someone skilled at driving with a manual shifting car, hardly thinks about pressing the gas pedal, clutch or manually moving the stick when shifting. Sometimes our ability to multitask with implicit memory is referred to as second nature because it is taking place without full awareness. But really, it would be better referred to as first nature since these actions from the old brain are taking place almost automatically and most often prior to our *consciously* thinking about them. In other words, we take actions or have behavioral reactions without intentionally or consciously making the decision.

Other types of automatic governing and behaviors that arise from *amygdala*, include reactive emotions like uncontrollable anger, rage, fear, pleasure, excitement and even uncontrollable joy. This is the area of the brain where our survival mode and inspiration or motivation originate. It is the location in brain of uncontrollable behaviors like addiction, road rage, anxiety disorders, obsessive compulsive disorder (OCD) and post-traumatic stress disorder (PTSD). As an unconscious, autopilot function, the amygdala stimulates the secretion of hormones that regulate heart rate, blood flow and dilation of the pupils. Highly important in the process of slowing or preventing healing, implicit memory is also the place where beliefs and judgements are processed, stored and expressed. This includes limiting beliefs and thoughts about illness and health that may not be true. It is from this deep-seated implicit memory that we have reactive behaviors defending untrue beliefs and ideas concerning illness and healing. From this area of the brain, we have a prefixed beliefs or ideas about illness, such as, regarding the way we *think* we are supposed to be treated, how an illness will progress and what the outcome will be. Those thoughts being limiting or positive and optimistic, whether true or not, will have great impact on the degree and permanence of healing.

"Trying" to be Conscientious...

With an understanding of how thoughts are processed and stored in the brain, the reason is revealed for why, "trying so hard to heal" may not achieve the desired results. The problem is, *procedural memory* (the Old Brain/subconscious mind) is a million times stronger than *declarative memory* (prefrontal cortex/conscious mind). In other words, the unconscious mind, the one that works on autopilot, is a million times stronger than the conscious, logical, thinking mind. That being the case, as conscious and conscientious as we can possibly be regarding illness and health, our declarative memory makes up only 10% of our thoughts and behaviors. These conscious thoughts and behaviors are constantly competing with the autopilot, over-ridding influences of the subconscious mind and procedural memory. We are most often guided by the automatic thinking, reactions and behaviors from our procedural memory, our subconscious mind. Meaning we primarily function from old, well-practiced knowledge, understanding and beliefs that may not only be inaccurate, but regularly justifying established limiting thoughts and barriers to healing.

This is the reason that conscious, conscientious people dealing with illness can easily from their explicit memory in the prefrontal cortex, say something like, "I believe in my doctor, I trust in the treatment, I believe I am healing and in perfect health." They truly, consciously believe that to be true. At the same time though, their implicit memory in the old brain, the subconscious mind, the one with the deeply fixed memories, limiting beliefs and judgements, is sabotaging that truth. The subconscious mind is instead, saying something like, "Nope, not true, nice try, you don't really believe that..." As I previously pointed out, this "trying so hard" to believe, most often turns out to be simply *wishing and hoping.* The conscious mind having surrendered to a more deeply embedded footprint of what we truly believe. In other words, our subconscious mind over-rides the cognizant, thinking mind, with well-defined patterns of automatic behaviors and reactions to illness and health, originating from the childhood development of our healing consciousness.

Reformatting healing consciousness is in some way, part of your current practice as a physician, healer and in self-healing. In this book, we are learning and expanding ways for modifying our own implicit memory, and that of patients and clients. One of the goals towards alter healing consciousness is by over-ridding the current, permanent, automatic and limited thinking around illness and health. We want to replace limiting implicit memories, with new permanent, automatic improved memories, ones with better knowledge and understanding related to the unlimited possibilities in healing. The intention is to reprogram old thoughts, beliefs and behaviors in our self, in patients and recipients of healing, thereby opening the door to triggering the body's natural ability to heal itself without old barriers and limitations.

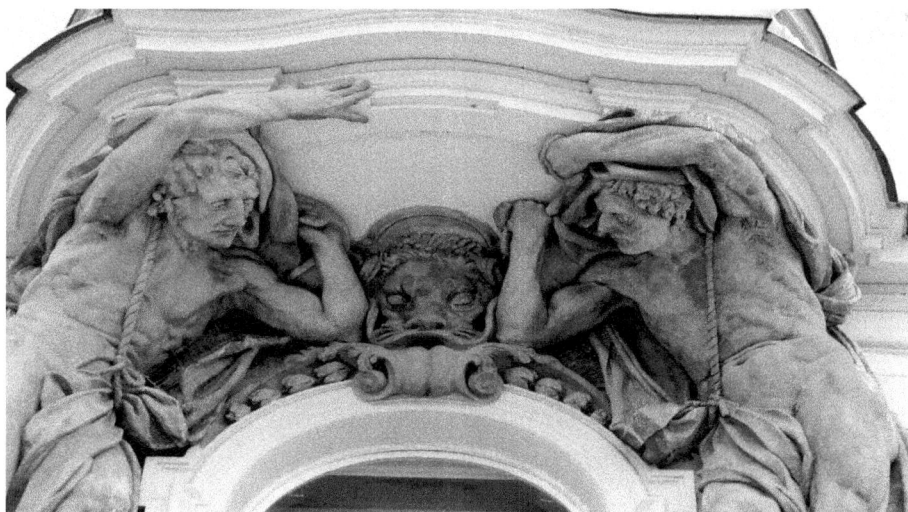

CHAPTER FIVE

Stress And Disease

B efore moving onto the tools and practices for aligning the five essential components for healing, another important disease generating force needs to be addressed in some detail. *Persistent physical and emotional stress* not only cause disease, but delay recover, prevent complete healing and build barriers to improving health. Studies show that thoughts and feelings in the form of anger, resentment, aggression, low self-esteem, rejection and other feelings resulting from social distress, not only cause physical pain and depression, but also produce objective physical and emotional disease. At minimum, these feelings can aggravate or prevent the immune system and healing process from functioning efficiently.

Every thought and emotion, positive or negative, triggers anatomical and physiological biochemical reactions that either move the body in a rebalancing, healing direction, or towards dysfunction and disease. A recent study by lead researcher and professor of psychology at Ohio State, Barbara L. Andersen, revealed that reducing stress in cancer patients not only improved mood and quality of life, but slowed progression of cancer, reduced recurrence of breast cancer and improved outcomes overall. I cannot stress enough, how our body reacts to every thought, feeling and emotion, even to the point of permanently altering our genetic coding. It is easier to understand how our genes are affected and altered by outside forces, such as, the food we eat, water we drink and by the air we breathe. But, the power of our thoughts, feelings and emotions are even more potent instruments in permanently modifying our DNA. This is the field of *Epigenetics*, described as the manner which our DNA is affected and altered by outside forces. As epigenetic influencers, emotional conflicts, guilt, shame, anger, resentment and joy, all stimulate and alter our anatomy and physiology. Some of these responses and modifications take place in the forms of increased heart rate, rapid blood flow, variations in of our breathing, digestion, changes in nervous system function and stimulation or suppression of the immune system. Other reactions include alteration in hormonal function, stimulation of glands and organs, modification of every aspect of our biochemistry and ultimately modifying our health on the cellular level.

While I believe it to be a bit more complex, a large population of doctors and psychologists consider most all cancers the result of emotional states of being. These professionals also believe that illness develops from alterations in our body resulting from life-trauma, chronic stress, anger, resentment, negativity, unre-solved conflict, feelings of unworthiness and low self-esteem. They have outlined different types of "cancer personalities." This group of healthcare professionals believe that treatment for cancer should be targeted not only at the physical disease, but also for the emotional basis for its cause.

There are a wide variety of health conditions more typically associated with stress and negative states of being, including obesity, heart disease, Alzheimer's disease, depression, diabetes, high blood pressure, increased cholesterol, insomnia, dementia, headaches, anxiety, phobias, stomach and intestinal conditions, joint pain, asthma, accelerated aging and cancer. Emotional stress is known to trigger an acute heart attack. Stress significantly disrupts the body's ability to regulate inflammation, stimulate the immune system, the hormonal system, will disrupt digestive function and promote the development or progression of many diseases. Stress is not the only emotion that causes changes in the body. Literally every thought we have generates a reaction and modification in our body on a gross, cellular and genetic level.

What is stress anyway? In simple terms, a book definition would be something along the lines of, "a state of physical, mental, emo-tional strain or tension, resulting from adverse or demanding cir-cumstances." In other words, stress is caused by how we are thinking and interpreting situations in life. Based on these effects of stress-ful thoughts, we can then understand how emotional and physical illness can be caused by the way we are thinking. Stress is an inside job, related to our own unique life perspective. Whether referring to a friend, a boss, finances or any other life situation, we create our own outlook and reality. One might have a positive, uplifting, inspiring perspective of a person or situation, while someone else might choose to see the same person or situation from a negative and suppressive perspective. As an example, consider two employees working for the same manager. One individual is resentful, complaining about how mean, unkind and hard driving the boss is, while the other person likes the same supervisor, finding them focused, challenging and effective. Positive thoughts and emotions lead to positive healthy changes in the body and mind, while the negative perspectives create unhealthy changes and illness.

Stress is created by *the way we think*. Over time, stress can cause undesirable, permanent changes in our genetic coding and ultimately our health. Thoughts trigger feelings and emotions. You might have noticed that when you are under stress, you are more susceptible to confusion, poor decisions, colds, flus and sickness. Coming down with a flu or infection rarely results solely by way of germs passing from one person to the next and is instead, part of a bigger picture most always including physical and/or emotional stress. On the rare occasion I have a cold or flu, there is always a direct correlation to my doing too much, burning the candle at both ends, not getting enough rest or been dealing an overwhelming amount of physical or emotional stress. Living in unhappy, negative thoughts and feelings will eventually lead to ill- health.

The immune system and the body's ability to regulate inflammation are seriously compromised by emotional stress and anxiety. Research tells us that the anti-inflammatory properties of the body have a direct, symbiotic relationship with the immune response. When inflammation is present, there is an increase in production of white blood cells (lymphocytes, T-cells, B-cells, macrophages, leukocytes) necessary for fighting infection and healing. This relationship is disrupted when we are under emotional stress. We become more susceptible to illness and less able to fight disease in the body. With prolonged over-activation of the immune system due to even mild chronic illness or ongoing life stress, the body may begin attacking itself, setting off an autoimmune response. In other words, the body begins to see its own tissues as pathology and attacks or in some way injures itself.

Cortisol and Illness

One important factor associated with stress initiating illness through the energy of thoughts and emotions, are chronically elevated levels of cortisol circulating in the body. Cortisol is often referred to as "the stress hormone," as if it is cortisol causing us stress. This is an unfair labelling of cortisol as it is a highly important hormone for the body. Produced in the *adrenal glands* (adrenal cortex), which sit atop the kidneys, cortisol is injected into the bloodstream as a response to physical or mental stresses. It is the hormone that during an emergency, enables what is referred as the "fight or flight reaction." Cortisol is also released into the bloodstream when there are low levels of glucose (sugar) in the body, aiding in the metabolism of fat, protein and carbohydrates. Cortisol is also the body's most effective temporary anti-inflammatory and pain reliever. The prescription anti-inflammatory medication, *cortisone*, is modeled after the natural cortisol hormone. Additionally, cortisol is important in stimulating glucose levels in the blood and within muscles. This generates a rush of energy in the body by stimulating the release of epinephrine (aka: adrenaline), boosting strength and physicality in response to an urgent situation.

Problems develop, though, when there are chronically elevated levels of cortisol circulating in the bloodstream. Normally, as a result of inflammation in the body from stress or illness, cortisol is designed to be released into the bloodstream reducing that inflammation. When the inflammation responds properly and diminishes, the production and release of cortisol is also supposed to stop and be resorbed. But too often this is not the case. Rather than an end in production or resorption of the circulating cortisol, in an attempt by to the body to maintain homeostasis, decides it is normal to have persistent, chronic elevation of cortisol in the bloodstream. Not exclusive to cortisol, the body commonly adapts to prolonged levels circulating chemicals in the bloodstream. For example, when anti-inflammatory medication is taken over prolonged periods, while initially effective, the body will eventually adapt to the drug, consider the inflamed tissues normal and result in the medication no longer being affective. The same is true for persistently elevated levels of cortisol. Over time the tissues become desensitized, whereby the anti-inflammatory and pain-relieving properties become ineffective. Pain and inflammation instead, not only remain, but worsen over time, becoming chronic. The problem with chronic inflammation is that it leads to other forms of disease and illness.

Cortisol combined with the neurotransmitter adrenaline (epinephrine), are injected into the bloodstream when there is an extreme emergency. This is what allows us to perform tasks that might typically seem impossible, like the stories we hear of someone lifting a car off their child. When cortisol is increased in the circulatory system, blood vessels constrict (get narrower), the heart-rate increases, muscles are tensed, blood pressure is elevated, respiration (breathing) becomes more rapid, the immune system is depressed, digestion suppressed, and the brain moves from creative cognitive thinking to more narrowly focused thoughts and movements. These actions within the body are all focusing awareness only on what is immediately necessary to survive. Cortisol is meant to be a short-term biochemical surge into the blood in order to deal with an urgent situation. Once the emergency has passed, cortisol is supposed to diminish until required again.

When chronic levels of elevated cortisol or inflammation are persistent in the body, illness and disease will result. One problem is that physical and mental dangers are not the only stresses increasing cortisol levels in the bloodstream. Many of what we consider normal daily activities, create enough stress to produce a regular production of cortisol. It is easy to understand the process of cortisol being boosted in the blood when we are being chased by a tiger in the jungle, and that when the danger has passed, the cortisol level also retreats. In our daily reality, most people living in these busy times have many life situations that create persistent levels of chronic stress with varying degrees of intensity. Stress can be found in the workplace, in relationships, around money, family, raising children, careers, school, marriages, associated with siblings, parents, mortgages, and the list being endless. These stresses create persistent elevated levels of cortisol circulating throughout the body that rarely, if ever, have a chance to abate. It is not uncommon in our daily lives that the body thinks and functions as if on high alert, as if it is in a state of almost constant urgency or emergency. Chronic stress, elevated cortisol and inflammation are significant factors in delaying or limiting the body's ability to heal, while reducing our capacity to reformat healing consciousness and align the five essential components for healing.

Physical Changes in the Body When Cortisol Levels Are Elevated

Due to the importance of understanding the effects of cortisol on our ability to heal ourselves and others, following is a list of the some of the physical changes taking place in response to an emergency. These are the same physiological effects occurring in the body any time there are chronically elevated levels of circulating cortisol. They are the same affects that result from prolonged, everyday life stress:

1. Epinephrine (adrenaline) is injected into the bloodstream.
2. Respiration increases (rapid shallow breathing).
3. Heart rate and cardiovascular system tension are increased.
4. Blood pressure is elevated.
5. Creative, cognitive thinking is placed on hold, being replaced by more immediately focused and urgent thoughts.
6. The immune system is depressed reducing the body's ability to heal itself.
7. Digestion is suppressed, causing a disturbance nutrient absorption.
8. Vasoconstriction (narrowing of blood vessels) in the vascular system.
9. Blood cholesterol levels are elevated.
10. Ability to sleep is disrupted.
11. The reproductive system is repressed, reducing proper function.
12. Calcium uptake in the intestine is reduced, affecting bone density.
13. Collagen synthesis and bone formation are inhibited, reducing healing in soft and bony tissues.
14. Wound healing is slowed.
15. Sodium is retained in the soft tissues.
16. Muscles become tense.

Think about the example of being chased by a tiger in the jungle where the body is only interested and focused on survival, not being injured or killed. Our body is not concerned with trying to heal a cut on a finger or cure cancer, so it suppresses the immune. It also cares not about digesting our last meal or whether an egg might be fertilizing and implanted in the reproductive system, thereby repressing the digestive tract and reproduction abilities. In a state of emergency, our mind is not trying to be creative or having intellectual epiphanies. Instead our thoughts are solely concentrated on where we will take our next step in fleeing or placing our hands in combat, protecting ourselves and families.

When daily activities are filled with stressful situations, whether extreme or mild, there is a continuous flow of cortisol circulating throughout the body. This chronic level of cortisol throughout the system can trigger the malfunction of most every cell and organ in the body, eventually leading to ill-health. Chronically elevated cortisol in the bloodstream suppressing our immune system, seriously reduces its ability to protect and heal our body. With daily stress maintaining elevated levels of cortisol, promoting persistent, widespread inflammation in the body, it is not surprising that many diseases once considered rare are now becoming commonplace.

Understanding the effects of stress and cortisol, it is no wonder there are so many patients suffering from digestive problems, bowel and bladder issues lining the waiting rooms of doctors' offices. This is associated with suppression of digestive tract function, from chronically elevated blood levels of cortisol. Further, when gastric and intestinal tract suppression occurs due to the increase in cortisol and epinephrine, there is a reduction in nutrient absorption by the gastrointestinal tract, even if we are eating healthfully. That feeling of "butterflies" in the stomach, often associated with being excited or nervous, can be a sign that the stomach is in a state of tension that will reduce its ability to digest and assimilate foods.

A common scenario for eating goes something like this, the average person sits down to eat a meal, ideally not fried, processed or fast foods. They eat as if having a shovel in each hand stoking the furnace of a locomotive and continue to stuff themselves until they can hardly breathe. A short time later, when feeling somewhat less full (not necessarily hungry), they eat until feeling full again. This process repeats itself throughout the day. By the end of a day, while they have eaten a large quantity of food and feeling almost constantly full, they are at same time, somehow still hungry. Even though they have eaten volumes of food, their body may still not have received the necessary nutrients required. And the process begins again the following day. This is part of the reason society overall has been getting larger and less healthy. Part of the problem in over-eating, might be in the body striving to obtain the required nourishment from nutrient poor foods. On the other hand, if our digestive system is not functioning properly due to excessive levels of stress and elevated cortisol, we would also need greater volumes of food, in an effort to gain the required daily nutrients for optimal function and healing.

Also, when cortisol and epinephrine levels are elevated in the blood, glucose (sugar) production is increased from the liver. This increase in blood sugar is designed to give a short-term energy boost when dealing with that emergency. But when no emergency exists, and sustained levels of cortisol are being caused by chronic, low-grade, daily stress making it difficult for blood glucose to be utilized, the body becomes vulnerable to conditions, such as, diabetes and obesity (the sugar storing in tissues as fat).

On a short technical note for those interested, cortisol is controlled by the hypothalamus (a small area of the brain) which releases a hormone CRR (corticotropin releasing hormone), triggering release of another hormone, ACTH (adrenocorticotropic hormone) from the pituitary gland (at the base of the brain). Together, when these hormones are discharged into the bloodstream, they reach the adrenal glands, stimulating the production of more cortisol and other steroidal hormones which in-turn, increase blood cholesterol levels. The result being a cyclic pattern of elevated hormones that can lead to many different types of illness, including cardiovascular disease, diabetes, obesity and emotional distress syndromes.

Following here are six steps for the healthiest way to eat and live in maintaining ideal health, longevity, to be trim and physically fit. These six mindful concepts promote the reformatting for your healing consciousness and aid in aligning the five essential components for healing. If you follow these six steps, your body will have the greatest opportunity to absorb and assimilate the nutrients necessary for being vibrant, healthy, creative, efficient, expansive and joyful. Additionally, by following these guidelines, you will never have to go on another diet. I will focus more on the first four *secrets to health, longevity and fitness,* as greater detail is given for secrets five and six in the following chapter presenting exercises and practices.

The Six Secrets to Health, Longevity and Fitness

1. Eat Close to The Farm.
2. Create A Pleasant Eating Environment.
3. Mindful Eating.
4. Conscious Eating.
5. A Daily Practice of Mindfulness.
6. Daily Movement and Exercise.

1. *Eating Close to the Farm* in simple terms means eating only *whole foods*. Eat nothing processed, especially avoid refined sugar. This means little to no restaurant food, which at best, is hardly ever simple or whole, even in healthy restaurants. Besides restaurants overusing sodium and sugar, even menu items as simple as salads and vegetables fail to report the contents of dressings, sauces and types of oils used for cooking. The concept is to predominantly eat fresh fruits, vegetables, grains, fish and meats that you prepare and cook yourself. Ideally using organic foods, though whole foods in any form, organic or not, will be healthier than processed foods. While the word *natural* alone means nothing on foods, it is possible to buy more reasonable priced products that have been grown and processed in the same way as their "certified" organic counterparts. These products branded as natural, will have labels clearly identifying commonly found organic food features, such as, non-GMO, no hormones, no antibiotics and no pesticides. Some farmers and processers want to avoid spending the money and time jumping through federal guideline hoops in order to gain official USDA organic certification. Some non-certified natural growers may follow even stricter guidelines than is required for gaining an organic designation. The key here is, eating *close to the farm* and whole foods at

home, providing control over knowing exactly what you are eating and how your body, mind and soul are being nourished.

2. *Eating in a Peaceful Environment.* Avoid eating while talking on the phone, scanning social media or searching the Internet. Steer clear of most reading and all television while eating. If you choose to read, make it something funny or spiritually enhancing. Ideally, eat with people you enjoy being with and keep the conversation to pleasant subjects. No politics, religion or war. Any activities while eating, reduces our presence to the meal and creates varying degrees of tension in the stomach and gastrointestinal tract. Actively doing something other than being present to eating and creating a pleasant environment, disrupts the body's ability to digest and assimilate the needed nutrients.

3. *Mindful Eating* includes having an appreciation or gratitude for the food on our plate, sincerely savoring the flavors, fully chewing all foods we ingest and enjoying the process. Having a grateful thought, saying *grace* or doing a short meditation of thanks can be a pleasant way to become present to a meal and begin mindful eating. We take the process of food, its preparation and eating for granted. It seems so simple, going to the market, shopping for food, putting it in a pot and having a meal show up on our plate. But if we thought about what it takes for a single vegetable to find its way to a supermarket shelf, we might see it as drop-to-your-knees magical. Think for a moment, about the amount of people it took to harvest the seed, transport the seed to market, sell the seed to growers at the right time of year, the farmers and workers growing the food, harvesting, packaging the foods and selling to a market. Then, all those who load, unload and transport the foods to buyers then stores, the ones that stock the

shelves before we make our purchase and those who check us out at the register. Domestication of the foods we eat today developed over thousands of years by skilled farmers and scientists, employing the brilliant sunshine, magnificent volumes of water and workers operating machinery. Our ability to buy an orange in most cities around the world, let alone volume of foods available to us from the synchronization of man and nature is nothing short of a miracle. There is so much to feel a grateful for, so many reasons to appreciate every bite of food we take.

Once we have food on our plate, it is not uncommon for people to eat quickly without awareness and tasting only the first bite or two. They follow those first tastes with an unconscious shoveling of food into their mouths like stoking a that train engine with coal, barely chewing and sometimes practically swallowing their food whole. This results in missing the unique, delicious flavors and joy in eating whole foods. Most people have forgotten how natural foods taste with the incessant heaps of salt, sauces and seasonings. In mindful eating, we look at what we are going to put in our mouths, noticing the color, texture, temperature and aroma. We fully chew every bite of food, making it more nutrient rich, more easily digestible and thoroughly tasting all the flavors. If you want to experience a new adventure in health and eating, feeling good and being highly productive, eat only whole foods that you cook at home for four weeks. Avoid salt, sugar and eat in a peaceful environment, chewing your foods well, enjoying all their beautiful and natural flavors.

4. In step four, practicing *Conscious Eating* alludes to having awareness of the *state* of our body and mind while eating. In this practice, we have awareness of when our body needs nutrients and when that need has been satisfied. This type of body awareness will prevent us from overeating. Conscious Eating means that we

begin eating when we are truly hungry and not just because we are bored or because it is dinner hour. We eat mindfully, not hurriedly. A meal is not something we are trying to *get out of the way*, it is to nourish the body and enjoy. With conscious eating, there comes a point during a meal where we no longer have feelings of hunger. In that awareness, we recognize our body and mind being are fully nourished and in need of no more food regardless of what might be remaining on our plates. Not surprisingly, this feeling of being satisfied might take place only one quarter or a third of the way through a typical serving. It is much easier to sense our body having had enough food if we are eating intentionally, slowly and consciously.

So far in this step, we have only eaten because we were hungry and have awareness that our body has had enough food. At this point, the body has been nourished, had adequate food for functioning healthfully and efficiently. The next step in conscious eating is to let it be okay to stop eating. Wrap up the food and save it for later when your body is hungry again. Too often people are eating just to "clear their plate" as told in childhood, "There are people starving in the world." Just as often, we might continue to eat *socially*. This refers to mindless eating when accompanied by others. In this scenario, as longs as there is food on the table and others are eating, we also continue to eat. Even long after the awareness of our body being satisfied and may even prefer not to eat anymore. Getting up from a social meal, many people realize they have unconsciously overeaten and are completely stuffed.

Another reason people overeat during or between meals is not because they are hungry, but rather out of boredom. When we feel bored, emotional or sad, we might attempt to gain comfort and joy through eating tasty foods. If we are consciously eating, we realize that feeling good from food would only last for a minute or two. The key is to maintain awareness of our body and mind anytime we are eating. If we are truly feeling and listening to our body related to food, it will always tell us when it is hungry, nourished, satisfied, comfortable and happy. I will repeat it again because it's important, feeling nourished and sated at a meal will always take place long before we feel full or our plate is empty.

5. The fifth step, having a *Mindful Practice*, might be described as an exercise in expanding awareness of our physical and mental state. It is an awareness of how our perception of the world interacts and relates to physical reality. While people commonly associate a mindful practice with meditation, it might also include any quiet time where we observe ourselves as if from the outside looking in, focusing on how our body, mind and emotions, interrelate with the people and the world around us. A mindful practice can take place on quiet stroll or hike communing with nature, in the shower or bath, in breathing exercises, active / passive relaxation, playing a musical instrument, mindful listening of music or chanting. A mindful practice might take place while in service to others. As with meditation, any of these activities can include a mantra, a specific intention or a desire, such as, harmony or healing. A daily meditation practice, having some silence and quiet time is a powerful mindfulness tool. They are instruments for becoming more centered, calm, intuitive and empowered. In the following chapter, I give detailed instructions in a variety of simple meditation practices.

6. *Daily Movement and Exercise*, the last of the six steps. Losing weight cannot be accomplished by following a diet alone. The body through homeostasis, will always work toward its own idea of a comfortable weight based on history of physical conditioning. To loose weight, exercise is essential for increasing metabolism. When

we move our bodies, there are the obvious benefits of exercise, like strengthening muscles and joints, burning calories, losing weight, becoming more toned and improving cardiovascular health. But there are other benefits of regular exercise that are important to reducing stress and elevated cortisol. Science tells us that exercise will increase our energy, strengthen bone density, improve memory, boost cognitive thinking, reduce the risk of chronic disease and increase joy in one's life. Exercise is also a mood booster, improving sleep, promoting a better sex life, reducing pain and increasing life span. Daily exercise can be in the form of walking, swimming, running or dancing, depending on your health and ability. Ideally, we exercise as vigorously as we can without injuring ourselves, which typically changes the type of activities we participate in with age. We want to avoid activities that might result in overexertion or injury. Based on a person's health, at least twenty minutes of exercise a day would be highly beneficial. While not practical for many people, building up to 60 minutes a day of exercise would be even better. If you have not been exercising regularly, begin a daily routine with short periods, slowly adding small amounts of time and effort each week. Depending on age and physical conditioning, some people may not be able to exercise for the suggested twenty minutes. More important, will be to exercise within safety and comfort, even if only five or ten minutes a day. If you are unsure of your conditioning and the types of exercise that best benefit you, consult with your doctor and seek guidance of a trainer.

Those are the six secrets to health, longevity and fitness. Practicing each one, enhances and expands your healing consciousness toward greater possibilities in healing. Combined with the practices and exercises presented in the coming chapter, will advance your skills at intentionally and purposefully aligning the five essential components for healing yourself and others. And now let us return to the subject of how stress and cortisol cause disease and prevent healing.

We know that stress and elevated levels of cortisol disrupt the reproductive system. While youth in the past were frequently taking measures to avoid getting pregnant, a serious change in that regard has arisen over the last decade or two. Millions and millions of couples have been struggling to become pregnant. They have found themselves resorting to medically assisted pregnancy through artificial insemination and laboratory in-vitro fertilization. Infertility has become a serious health problem, especially in the United States, where 2016 recorded the highest rates of infertility in the last 100 years. A recent study in Canada revealed that in 1984, there were 5.4 million invitro fertilizations and in 2011, 15.7 million medically-assisted fertilizations. Additionally, there has been a trend in low birth weight babies. A review of 185 studies, reveal a 59.3% drop in the sperm count and quality of sperm in men between 1973 and 2011 in North America, Australia and New Zealand.

While there are many theories surrounding low sperm counts, chemicals, pesticides, alcohol, smoking, radiation and stress are typically at the top of most lists. I would add to the list, the air we breathe, but place an emphasis on chronic levels of stress. These reasons for reducing sperm count have been called environmental castration. Chronic stress, chronic levels of elevated cortisol in men, can disrupt testosterone production, sperm production, can cause erectile dysfunction and be associated with an enlarged prostate gland.

For women, stress and chronic levels of elevated cortisol can create irregular menstrual cycles, stop the cycle completely or lengthen them time between periods, making impregnation difficult. With stress, women might experience more painful menstruation, retain more fluids, suffer from bloating and have drastic mood swings. The most common physical cause of infertility in women is polycystic ovaries, a condition where there are multiple, fluid filled cysts on the ovary, reducing their ability to function properly. But what causes polycystic ovaries? Just as in men, women are exposed to stress, elevated cortisol levels and the same environmental factors listed above, all contributing to infertility. Chemicals in plastics, the most notable being Bisphenol A (BPA), are not examined and discussed often enough. BPAs and similar chemicals have been used in plastic for baby bottles, cookware, water bottles, food storage, zip lock bags, plastic eating ware and thermal paper since the 1950s. These BPAs exhibit estrogen, hormone-like properties that since 2008 have been known to create serious and chronic illness. Yet it wasn't until 2012 after 70 years of regular use in our food products that the EPA banned the use of BPAs, but only in baby bottles. They are known to disrupt endocrine (hormone) balance, affecting the ovaries, sperm count and fertility. While health risks associated with BPAs remain a topic of scientific debate, after seven decades of use, the European Chemical Agency has listed the substance, as "very high concern due to its properties as an endocrine disruptor." There has also been a trend in the healthy products industries where they have stopped using plastics with BPAs for water bottles and eating utensils. The problem remains, as the replacement for non-BPA plastic products appear to have similar effects on the body and are not a healthier alternative. Another modern era concern being researched for its effects on fertility is the *electromagnetic fields* associated with electronic equipment, such as, computers, cellphone and home electronics. While the evidence for impact on health by low dose electrical field emissions from these products is currently not very strong, like plastics, it might take many decades of use and study to fully understand their impact disease.

We know that chronic levels of stress and increased circulating cortisol levels can inhibit fertility and reduce sexual desire in both men and women. Additionally, they can have lasting effects on a fetus, including lower birth weight, emotional consequences, impact on brain development and potential behavior. Current statistics tell us that 40% of couples will have difficulty becoming pregnant annually, totaling about 7.4 million women in America.

Being in a consistent state of low-level stress, being on edge, with persistently elevated levels of cortisol, keeps the entire body in a constant state of tension and distress, as if always ready to take care of an emergency or urgent situation. The body is then in a relentless state of trying to create homeostasis and balance, eventually giving up and allowing that elevated levels of stress hormone to be considered normal. Another adverse effect of elevated cortisol are chronic pain syndromes, such as, often mis-diagnosed chronic fatigue syndrome. Prolonged elevation of cortisol also leads to muscle wasting, reduces calcium uptake in the intestines, inhibiting bone formation and thereby contributing to osteoporosis. The amount of calcium we ingest in foods will not off-set the fact that the calcium is not being absorbed by the gastrointestinal tract due to elevated levels of cortisol. Collagen synthesis, important for building and repairing connective tissues, skin, muscles and tendon is reduced, thereby inhibiting and suppressing normal healthy tissue regeneration. This causes an acceleration of tissue aging, increased susceptibility to injury, while slowing tissue recovery when damaged. Elevated cortisol and epinephrine, slow wound healing and promote sodium absorption and retention in the blood and tissues, this in turn, can lead to hypertension, heart disease and many other health issues.

Additionally, when chronically elevated cortisol and stress are present, cognitive and creative thinking are almost completely suppressed, replacing or eliminating our ability to have imaginative, logical, productive and mindful thoughts. Only the most urgent thoughts for survival remain present. The quick, short-term emergency thinking, in-the-moment thoughts, operating only to protect and defend, while inhibiting memory storage and retrieval. Because of the cellular urgency taking place, meaning every cell of the body is on high alert, insomnia is another common symptom of stress and elevated cortisol.

There is a normal course the body goes through processing and eliminating cortisol and epinephrine from our system. It is part of maintaining homeostasis and an unending effort towards generating optimal health. Every cell of the body has glucocorticoid receptors that receive cortisol. These receptors located in chromosomes (location of genetic information) of the nucleus (the control center) are designed to bring the hormone into the cell where it activates specific functions. In addition to previously described functions of cortisol, these actions also include, speeding up or slowing down metabolism, stimulating nutrient processing and maintaining homeostasis. Once the cortisol has been utilized by the cell, it is broken-down and eliminated. The system fails when cells of the body are overwhelmed with more cortisol then they have the capability to use, resulting from over production or lack of elimination. This creates the chronically elevated levels of cortisol circulating throughout the body, eventually creating biochemical imbalances and opening the door to the adverse effects of illness and disease.

Taming out-of-control, chronically elevated levels of cortisol in our body and calming chronic stress in our lives, we need to acquire exercises and habits that are calming, centering and mindful.

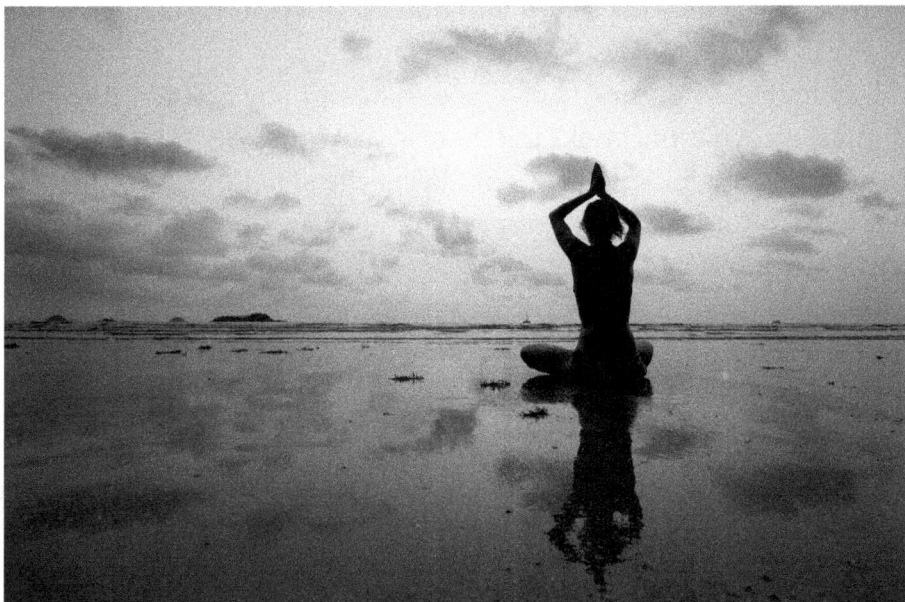

CHAPTER SIX

Exercises In Aligning The Five
Essential Components For Healing

With an understanding of the five secret components for healing and how they bring us to that place of knowingness, let us look at ways we can intentionally and purposefully, align these essential components for healing, creating more optimal health while at the same time boosting our ability to heal ourselves and others. In Western medicine, we know that physicians are trained to find *the* diagnosis, as if there is always only a single and simple possibility for any illness. They then administer what the books tell them is the most effective treatment in relieving, maintaining and/or curing the symptoms of a disease. This too often results in narrow-minded, by-the-book medicine, meaning precisely practicing protocols in one specific manner that was learned in school, according to *the books*. Based on longtime practical experience and research, by-the-book medicine in any field of healthcare or healing, will as often as not, fail to realize highly important, unique, individual and critical concerns contributing to disease or a delay in healing. By-the-book medicine not uncommonly leads to a misdiagnosis, prescribing of unnecessary tests or incorrect medications and treatment. By-the-book medicine will almost always fail to take into consideration not only the unique nature of an individual's current history, anatomy and physiology, but will also fail to uncover and recognize their distinctive healing consciousness. They will miss the all-important nature of the patient's knowledge and understanding of their condition, how they emotionally deal with illness, what kind of support they have in their lives and whether their overall life experience is positive and expansive or negative and constrictive. To be most effective in healing and healthcare, the practitioner gains a clear picture of the way each patient uniquely understands illness and how they *believe* healing is supposed to take place. Unfortunately, these characteristics are not part of by-the-book medical protocol as we learn in our studies. Once we understand these unique aspects of our patient/ recipient, we will be able to connect with that part of their health perspective, allowing us to modify their healing consciousness. We can then guide them towards aligning the five essential components for healing and permanently broaden their possibilities for how healing take can place. The point is to open the door in releasing or removing deeply seated, subconscious, learned beliefs, practiced blocks, barriers and obstacles that delay or prevent healing. At the same, we move the patient towards creating new, permanent, automatic thoughts, behaviors and actions, knowing they have the capability of healing in ways they never knew possible.

Following here, are exercises and practices I will describe and illustrate for aligning the five essential components for healing. Some are writing exercises, others mindfulness practices or physical activities. More specific and detailed instructions follow this list for each exercise and practice. In the clinical setting, I discuss all these exercises and practices with patients during a treatment or coaching session, giving all patients unique and specific home care instructions and homework based on their condition. The goal is to better understand their current state of healing consciousness, help in removing blocks and barriers while developing and accelerating their ability and skills in actively healing themselves and others.

In addition to reducing stress, anxiety and elevated cortisol levels, the following practices and exercises are designed to have you investigate your own perspectives on illness, healthcare and healing. This is an important step in your ability to understand and remove unhealthy blocks and barriers, repressive learned thought patterns that might be causing illness that slow or prevent the greatest possible healing. At the same time, these practices will open the door to expanding and reformatting your automatic thinking around illness and health, creating thoughts and feelings that automatically align the five essential components for healing. The resultant affect is in bringing your healing consciousness to that place of knowingness and triggering the body's most powerful and natural healing response. In other words, these exercises can be an important process in reformatting your healing consciousness in the healthiest possible manner. I highly recommend a daily practice of numbers 2, 3, 5 and 7, while utilizing the others on an as needed basis, which may be quite frequent.

The *Six Secrets to Health, Longevity and Fitness* shared in the previous chapter are components of, and complementary to the following exercises and practices. My intention is to present practical applications promoting a reduction of stress and anxiety, stimulate the immune system, lower elevated levels of circulating cortisol, while promoting optimal health and healing. Practicing these exercises will aid in broadening one's healing consciousness and most of all, in aligning the five essential components for healing.

1. Writing Exercises
    a. Journal the way you *feel* about your condition.
    b. Journal your *thoughts, feelings and emotions* regarding your prescribed treatment.
    c. Journal *feelings you have* about your doctors.
    d. Journal possibilities for *releasing fear* related to illness.
2. Mindful Practices
    a. *Meditation* practices
       Gratitude meditation.
       Mantra meditation.
       Walking meditation.
       Visual focus meditation.
       Sound meditation.
    b. Progressive active, passive relaxation.
    c. Body mind practices
3. Dream Journaling

4. Anger, Resentment and Forgiveness Exercise
5. Movement and Exercise
6. Healthful Eating
7. Sound Therapy
8. Stream of Consciousness Journaling
    a. Gratitude Journaling
9. Stress Reduction and Healing Through Intimacy

While it seems that some of these writing exercises might create negative thoughts and feelings, as you will see, this is not the case. The goal of journaling is in part, to look at and confront feelings we carry that inhibit our ability to feel free, joyful and to heal. Something akin to an ostrich pulling its head out of the sand and living life. When we face the reality of life difficulties we may unknowingly be carrying in our body and minds, acknowledging these life truths creates an opportunity to release them, freeing ourselves of inner obstacles for healing. These writing exercises are for you alone. Write honestly, freely and without overthinking or judgement of what it all means. Stream of consciousness writing. Write your truth. The exercises begin with four journaling assignments. The first three can be written in the same sitting. The fourth writing exercise will be described separately.

*"Writing, it's a ritual, and you need to be brave
and respectful and sometimes get out of the way of
whatever it is that you're inviting into the room."*

TOM WAITS, AMERICAN SINGER, SONGWRITER

1. Writing Exercises

A. Journal how you *feel* about your condition. Include,
How it makes you feel and details of what you think about the condition? Maybe it creates fear or feelings of frailty. Maybe you feel old, sick, depressed, helpless or you might have few feelings about it. Write all the feelings you carry in your body and mind around your condition.
What have you been told and what do you understand about your condition? Write it all down.
Once you have nothing left to journal on the subject and in order to release those unhelpful mindsets, write a note to yourself that, "Negative thoughts and feelings related to my condition are choices and not necessarily true. They are just feelings that I can release."
Lastly for this exercise, make a list of other perspectives and feelings you can choose that are positive and healing. Write, "I am no longer a slave to fearful thoughts or feelings around my condition. I see my body and mind in perfect health."

B. Journal *thoughts, feelings and emotions* regarding your prescribed treatment.
What is the recommended treatment and how do you feel about it?
Do you believe it to be the right treatment for you?

Have you discussed your feelings about the treatment with your doctor?

How do you *believe* your condition is supposed to progress, and how are you *feeling* about that?

Finally, to release those negative thoughts and feelings, triggering healing perspectives in the body and mind, make a list of possible pathways your condition could heal. List every possibility including those you might have believed unlikely or even impossible. Journal the best possible scenario for your healing and finish the list with, "I am in perfect health."

C. Journal how you *feel*, and what you *think* about your doctors. Do you feel like you have the best doctor? Maybe you think he or she is the best but do not like them.

Is it possible you feel you have no choice?

Write all your feelings about your doctors including all the things you like about them.

If you are lacking trust in your doctor, you can limit your ability to heal from an illness.

Once you have written all your feelings and discomforts around your doctors, realize you have other options for choosing doctors.

You are also able to change the way you will feel about them. Next, write down what conversations you can have with your doctor in a heart to heart talk regarding the way you are feeling about them and your illness. Make sure all your questions will be answered.

Ultimately you may find the need to consult with another practitioner.

Make a list of every possibility you have for either improving your confidence in your doctor or making a change.

D. Journal the *releasing fears.*

Write on the following: *If I didn't have this medical condition, what other fears do I have in my life?*

Like anger and resentment, fear can cause physical and emotional disease, creating blocks and barriers not only to healing, but to creating what you want in your life.

Write all you can on fear, acknowledging and bringing forward any fears that might be interfering with your health or quality of life. This will allow you to acknowledge and release those fears, clearing a broader path to health and greater life joy.

Know that fear is a *thought* that we choose.

Sometimes we use fear to be immobilized in the present moment rather taking an action we would like to avoid. We have the choice in any moment to have a different thought and feeling, a courageous thought and feeling.

Journal all the reasons you can think of for not feeling fearful. Be courageous in those thoughts and feelings.

Lastly, make a list of all the better thoughts and feelings you can choose to have in the same situations, rather than fear.

If you are unable to release your fears or feel saddened by this exercise, skip ahead in this chapter, you will find a *gratitude journaling* exercise. This will further expand your healing consciousness, lift your spirits and allow alignment of the five essential components for healing.

Each of these writing exercises by themselves and together, bring to the forefront of the mind, our fixed ideas about illness and healing. In other words, how we are understanding illness and the way we *believe* healing takes place. Some of that knowledge and understanding may be accurate and others inaccurate or simply narrow understandings that can inhibit, slow or prevent greater possibilities for healing. Gaining perspective on our healing consciousness through journaling these thoughts and feelings, allows us to remove, modify or at least set aside narrow mindedness in relation to how the body responds to treatment, as well as creating new paths for healing. We may have been told by doctors, family, friends or have read something telling us that due to our age or genetic make-up, there is only one inevitable path for responding to an illness. Science tells us this is no longer true, that health is more important than age and our genes don't control us. Healing can take place in so many ways we never thought possible or understood. The more we understand the effects of our healing consciousness on dis-ease, the greater the opportunity we have for creating more effective healing thought patterns.

2. Mindful Practices

Sign Out, Switch Off, Turn Within

That might sound like a 1960s New Age motto, but one of the best things you can do right now is to turn off your smartphone and put it somewhere out of reach. Turn off the television, shut down computer games, put away food you're eating out of boredom, stop all your obsessive or compulsive activities, especially if you are doing these activities to avoid engaging in something you really want or need to be doing. If those behaviors prevent you from having some daily quiet time, put them away. In other words, it is time to learn how to reduce your intake and overflow of the extraordinary volumes of external, unnecessary stimulation flooding your mind, body and spirit. It is time to be courageous, stepping into actions that move you in the direction of your meaning and purpose.

Everyone has some way of overwhelming themselves with activities they enjoy or pretending to be productive in order to avoid taking useful actions in their lives. These interests might include an unending pursuit of pleasure and gratification through activities, from shopping, eating, exercising, watching television, playing video games, cooking and reading to drugs or alcohol to name a few. Any activity that prevents taking necessary or desired life actions, any behaviors that get in the way of taking responsibility in life or pursuits that prevent quiet time, can bring us out of alignment with the five secrets to healing. Any of these activities can produce chronic stress and elevated levels cortisol in the body, keeping us on edge, keeping us anxious, while preventing desired life achievements and disrupting the healing process.

When we participate in mindful practices and exercises that align the five essential components for healing, we are reducing cortisol and stress in our body and mind. This chapter is dedicated to reducing these chronically elevated levels of stress, cortisol and epinephrine. One of the most effective methods for reducing anxiety, stress and cortisol, is to be more in harmony with life and connected to our authentic selves through a meditation practice. I recommend at minimum, one daily meditation practice, even if just for ten minutes.

"You should sit in meditation for twenty minutes a day –
unless you're too busy; then you should sit for an hour."
ST. FRANCIS DE SALES, 16TH/17TH CENTURY CATHOLIC BISHOP

A. Meditation Practice

Most people understand meditation as a tool for calming and relaxation. A practice for reducing stress and anxiety. But meditation has a far greater reach into our anatomy, physiology, emotional and physical state of balance. Science tells us that meditation improves our focus and concentration, increases self-awareness, improves sleep, digestion and slows aging. Meditation cultivates higher cognitive thinking, boosts memory, stimulates the immune system, strengthens cardiovascular health, reduces pain, depression, high blood pressure, irritable bowel syndrome and reduces elevated levels of cortisol in the body. Following an eight-week study of mindfulness practices at Harvard University, MRI scans revealed an increase in gray matter and a shrinkage of the amygdala in the brain. We learned earlier, that this is of shrinkage in the brain is where old fixed beliefs, fears, anxiety, addiction behavior and anger are stored and expressed. It is also where the response to stress originates. This may be the reason that people who meditate experience greater happiness, more joy and an increased sense of well-being. Meditation improves physical health, emotional well-being and spiritual connection. Not only will meditation be a key component in aligning the five essential components for healing, but also inspire us in achieving important life goals.

In Western society, people often think that meditation is some far-out spiritual practice for Buddhist monks who sit alone on a mountain top in the Himalaya Mountains, clearing the minds of all thoughts for days on end and without a need for food or water. For some of us, trying to clear our minds of all thoughts sounds quite impossible and intimidating. While there are Buddhist monks who practice meditation in a similar manner described, there are many forms of meditation available to practice, from the very simple to more complex and working meditations. There are meditations that use tools and implements, such as, candles, mandalas, bells or focusing on objects.

The easiest and most effective way to begin meditating might be by playing guided meditation recordings. There are many websites and smartphone apps that offer guided meditations, some by well-known spiritual leaders, authors and speakers, all of which can be very valuable and gratifying practices. I have a large library of guided meditations for healing specific conditions and diseases, in addition to specialized meditations for relaxation, releasing fears and building a meditation workshop. My favorite form of meditation besides quiet time in nature is not a mind clearing meditation at all, but instead a productive practice I call *working meditations*. Following here are a variety of meditations that can be easily practiced.

Daily Gratitude Meditation

This first meditation is a simple though powerful daily meditation practice. Experiencing gratitude is healing and there are so many reasons to be thankful and joyful in this life. Simply waking up healthy in the morning makes you are luckier than the millions of people who will be sick or die that day. With money in your wallet, you are more fortunate than ninety percent of people in the world. Having a bed to sleep in or food to eat makes you more fortunate than more than half the world. Practicing gratitude, releases anxiety, fear, negative thoughts and feelings of anger and resentment, significantly contributing to alignment of the five essential components for healing.

The gratitude meditation begins with an intentional and potent deep breathing practice that by itself could be considered a meditation. Deep breathing is calming to the body and mind, lowering blood pressure, releasing endorphins, detoxifying the body, while oxygenating all organ systems important for healing. Deep breathing stimulates the immune system, boosts energy and raises our sense of well-being. Additionally, this deep breathing exercise opens the mind, body and spirit to our daily meditation practice. Be patient and consistent when first starting to meditate, as it can take some time and diligence in developing an effortless daily practice. With regular practice, meditation can be accomplished in as few has five or ten minutes, though over time, people become so inspired by the benefits of meditation, many naturally increase their practice to twenty or thirty minutes a day.

To begin, sit with your hands in your lap, recline or lay comfortably on your back with your arms at your sides and close your eyes. Give yourself a few minutes to get quiet and become aware of your breathing, then proceed as follows:

Step 1. Breathing; Take four slow, deep Qigong breaths.
         A Qigong breath is inhaling, ideally through the nose, slowly and as deeply as possible, first filling the stomach, making a round Buddha belly and then filling the lungs last. While focusing on the rising and falling abdomen, hold the breath for as long as possible.

Step 2. Following each Qigong breath, make a Tummo exhale, accomplished by pursing your lips as if you are going to kiss the universe, then exhaling the longest, slowest stream of air you can possibly make.

Step 3. Once you have completed the four Qigong breaths with Tummo exhaling, begin this meditation by bringing to the forefront of your mind, each current, stressful event or situation in your life, the ones that may be taking control of your thoughts and actions. While this process may take a bit of time in your first couple of meditations, it well worth the effort. Identify the negative energy and stresses you may be carrying related to relationships, career, money, partners, children, parents and family. Any thoughts or situations that are creating stress in your life, bring them forward and acknowledge their presence.

Step 4. Next, holding at the forefront of your mind, every negative life issue large and small, imagine a set of shelves to your left where you will be setting those negative and stressful thoughts. As you think of each life situation, person or thing that creates stress or negativity, place them one at a time on the shelves to your left. You will leave them here to dwell on the shelves and be out of your mind, body and spirit.
All that stress and negativity can remain there, out of your thoughts, to be revisited at another time if necessary and when convenient.
Continue this process until there are no more negative thoughts or emotions in your mind and body. Be sure that there is not one negative thought or feeling left. Over time, this practice will get much easier and quicker.

Step 5. Then, imagine another shelf to your right. This time, you will recall everyone and everything you are grateful to have in your life. Take a few moments to feel gratitude and appreciation for all of those who you love, the people who raise you up and support your process. Feel gratitude for things you have, such as, a roof over your head, a refrigerator with food in it, good health, family and friends, take a few moments to enjoy them. You can be thankful for having eyes to see with, as not everyone has vision, thankful for ears to hear music and voices, thankful for hands to feel and grasp with and legs to walk. Be grateful for everything you have had up to this moment in your life, for everything you have presently, and be grateful for all that lies ahead.

Once you have acknowledged and been thankful, for the people throughout your life and things you have enjoyed, place them one at a time on the shelf to your right. They will always be available for you to re-experience, enjoy and appreciate any time you please, whether within or outside of your meditation.

Know that there will always be far more to be grateful for in life than there are situations that create stress. The more often you recognize the positive perspectives of your life and embrace an appreciation for all you have, the healthier and happier you will be.

Step 6. The gratitude meditation concludes with three long, slow, Qigong breaths as described in step 1 above, followed by Tummo exhales illustrated in Step 2.

Regularly experiencing gratitude, expands our healing consciousness and promotes alignment of the five essential components for healing.

Mantra Meditation

Meditation using a *mantra* is probably the most common meditation practice worldwide. The mantra is a distinct word, sound or phrase, which is repeated over and over, encouraging our mind to turn-off outside influences while focusing on a specific intention from within our authentic selves. Man-tra can be literally defined as *transporting the mind.* A mantra can be used for planting a *seed of intention* into our mind and spirit during our meditation. Silent repetition of a mantra in meditation, creates a rhythmic pattern of sound that is said to liberate the mind while at the same time forming a spiritual connection. Science has described the benefits of a mantra meditation to include, reducing anxiety, depression and stress, blocking the release of adrenaline and cortisol, slowing heart rate and lowering blood pressure, calming the mind, moving healing energy through the body and releasing fear and worry.

You can create your own mantra or choose from one of many thousands. A mantra can be as simple as, *I am*, referring to God, to the godliness within us or that place where we are connected to God. You might choose a Buddhist or Sanskrit mantra, some of the most common being *om*, the sacred sound/symbol representing the entirety of the universe, Divine energy or all knowledge. The Hindu So-*ham*, might be employed as a mantra, denoting, "I am," or *rama*, another name for God (ra = God/sun, ma = mother/moon), *yam*, as a mantra referring to, "the seed of the Divine" or "seed of *the* energy." A powerful mantra I like from a Deepak Chopra meditation is, *Shara vana ya*, which means, "My awareness is aligned with the creative power of the universe." Setting a seed of intention at the beginning of your mantra, can reveal guidance about a life issue that may show itself during or more likely immediately following the meditation. Contemporary mantras could be something like, "I am in perfect health," "the next step in reaching my goal reveals itself to me" or "I am loving awareness." A simple mantra may also be a single repeated sound, name or word from a prayer book, especially a word or phrase that carries special meaning for you.

To begin a mantra meditation, speak the mantra out loud two or three times to impress it on your memory. For the balance of the meditation, the mantra is repeated silently. Sit with your hands in your lap, recline or lay comfortably on your back with your arms at your sides and close your eyes. Give yourself a few minutes to get quiet and become aware of your breathing. If you become distracted throughout the meditation, by sounds around you or thoughts in your mind, simply refocus your attention back to repeating the mantra. It is that easy.

Step 1. Choose a mantra.
If you are seeking guidance or clarity from your meditation related to a specific subject, set an intention or goal and bring that intention to the forefront of your mind.

Step 2. Sit with your palms up in your lap, lying down or reclined with arms relaxed at your sides.
Close your eyes. Sounds of nature or meditation music may make it easier when you are new to meditating.

Step 3.   (Optional but recommended) Take three or four Qigong breaths and Tummo exhale as described in the first two steps of the gratitude meditation.

Step 4.   Bring your meditation intention to mind.
Begin chanting your mantra out loud a few times or until it feels natural and easy, transitioning to silent repetition. If you have a timer with a gentle bell or ringer, you might set it in the beginning for ten minutes and work your way up to twenty or thirty minutes. There is no time limit however, on how long you choose to meditate.

Step 5.   To close your meditation, release the mantra and refocus your awareness back to the room or space where you are sitting. While optional, I suggest taking two or three long, slow Qigong breaths with Tummo exhaling, while reconnecting with your surroundings.
When you are comfortable, open your eyes.

Walking Meditation

A *Walking Meditation* is lovely way to meditate especially if done on a trail in nature or, even more compelling, in a *labyrinth*. Dating back 5,000 years, people have used labyrinths for peaceful, intentional, mindful walks. They are sometimes referred to as *prayer walks*. A labyrinth is spiral pathway that at first glance looks like a maze. The difference between a labyrinth and a maze is that the labyrinth has no tricky barriers to negotiate, there is only one way in and one way out. Their unique design creates a walk that seems longer than they might appear and eventually leading to a center point. Labyrinths are typically designed outdoors though at times, inlaid into the floors of churches and spiritual centers. Their paths might be defined as mosaics in pavement, by blocks or natural stone, though, may also be simply drawn on any surface.

To practice a *walking meditation*, whether you are walking a labyrinth or walking in nature, there are three stages. The process for a walking meditation, innately advances the alignment of the five essential components for healing. Before starting, take a few quiet moments looking into yourself and choose an intention for your walk. The focus of your intention might be on healing a specific condition in yourself or someone else. It may be that you want answers to a question, the solution for a problem, have guidance in relation to career, family, relationships or issues with a friend. You might look for guidance in making a business decision, simply calm your busy mind, work on healing yourself, others or find inspiration for a project. When you walk the labyrinth or on a path in nature, you move slowly and deliberately, while remaining focused on the intentions during the three stages.

Stage I: In the first stage, you stand at the entrance to the labyrinth or trailhead in nature, with a healing intention for yourself, for others, or ask a question for which you seek an answer. This intention will be your mantra for walking the labyrinth to the center or to the halfway point of your walk-in nature.

Enter the labyrinth walking with sincerity and contemplation, repeating the intention to yourself.

Stage II: When you reach the center of the labyrinth or halfway point of a nature walk meditation, pause, open your heart to receiving the results of your meditation intention.

This is where you generate the healing you seek, the new insight or answer to a question. Through listening and mindful awareness, acknowledge that healing has already taken place, or the question has been answered. Allow yourself to receive answers and healing. Visualize in your mind's eye, yourself or others already healed. Here and acknowledge the answer to a question or see yourself already having accomplished a desired goal.

Spend at least a few moments or however long you please, enjoying your calm, connected inner peace at the labyrinth's center.

Open yourself to the gifts of gratitude and joy.

If you feel as though guidance has not been unfolding for you, there is no need to worry. It is not uncommon that answers from a working meditation appear on the walk back from the center or arise seemingly out of nowhere on a later day. You will eventually realize, possibly having an epiphany of some sort, when your healing or answer appears another day or time.

Stage III: Before leaving the center of the labyrinth for the walk back, set an intention to seal your healing or guidance within yourself.

This intention is one of visualizing the healing that has already taken place. In other words, if you had an intention of healing a specific illness, see in your mind's eye, those tissues or organs fully healed. If you sought guidance on the walk in, this time visualize clearly and in detail, the next step towards achieving your specific goal or see your intention completed already.

Your exit intention will be your mantra, or you can practice gratitude on your walk back.

Leaving the center of the labyrinth or starting back on your
nature walk, continue with sincere, deliberate walking.

Repeat your new affirming intention or gratitude practice,
sealing inside yourself, the gift of this meditation.

Enjoy the awareness, motivation or inspiration that has arisen.

Over the days following any meditation, new answers and guidance might arise in profound or subtle ways. If you were to journal
your experience of the walking meditation, expanded realizations
will likely arise regarding your intentions, along with metaphorical
symbolism as we find in dream interpretation.

Visual Focus Meditation

A *visual focus meditation* is a meditation involving an external
physical device. The object is a tool for tricking the mind into
being present to the moment. It is a tethering point for the mind,
keeping it from drifting off into thoughts and stories. There are
two forms of *visual focus*, also called *object meditation* or *open-
eyed meditation* that will be described here. First is meditation
using an inanimate object. We are inundated with so much visual
input throughout the day, often creating great amounts of tension
in our body and mind, while distracting us from looking inwards
and being mindful. This is an exercise in drawing our consciousness away from life's distractions, while releasing all that visual
tension and clutter in our lives. A visual focus meditation can bring
us into the present moment where all the magic of manifestation
and healing take place. In this type of object meditation, we choose

a target to observe and focus on, while the physical nature of the item being irrelevant. You might choose a stone, a flickering candle, a leaf, flower, piece of fruit or any other inanimate object. It is best to choose an object you have little attachment to, as part of the intention will be to avoid thinking about the object itself. The second type of visual meditation is performed with an object that we do have attachment too, often a spiritual attachment. Some use the photograph of a teacher or holy person. Others use crystals, photographs of loved ones, spiritual icons or any other object that brings feelings of peace, love, harmony and joy.

Step 1. Choose your object.

Step 2. Place the object on a table or altar just below eye level.

Step 3. Sitting with your hands in your lap, take three or four Qigong breaths with Tummo exhaling (optional though recommended), as in the gratitude meditation.

Step 4. Over the first ten to fifteen minutes, keep a soft focus on the object. Gaze (without squinting) at one area of the article, without focusing on any detail. The periphery of your visual field remains present, but out of focus.
Avoid focusing on the object. The meditation is not about the object.
Each time you have any thought, acknowledge the thought, release it from your mind and return to your soft focus on the object.
Notice any sensation in your body, such as, pain or discomfort, and release those feelings, returning to your soft focus on the object.

Relax your body and your eyes.

Continue releasing all thoughts from your mind and feelings, pain or discomfort you have in your body.

Step 5. Following the soft-focus period, releasing thoughts and physical feelings, bring the object into focus and describe it silently in your mind in the greatest detail possible. Observe every aspect of the object without attachment, how light falls on the object, is it dull or reflective, describe the shape of its borders, the colors, density, what it is made of and its textures.

As you move through this meditation, you will find that redundant and overwhelming internal dialogue of life calms down and may even disappear. Cares of the world are released and replaced by higher energy feelings of joy and inspiration.

Step 6. To close this meditation, make two Qigong breaths, as long and slowly as you possibly can, hold the breath for as long as you can, and make the longest, slowest possible Tummo exhale. As you are breathing, refocus your awareness back to the room or space where you sit. When you are comfortable, open your eyes.

For the visual meditation using a spiritual figure, follow steps 1 to 3 in the object meditation above.

Step 4. Choose a meditation intention.

In this case it may be to connect to your spiritual figure, to God or to your own spiritual center.

It may be to ask for guidance from this spiritual leader or God. You may want to focus on a healing intention.

Step 5. Focusing on the image, use your intention as a mantra throughout your meditation.

Step 6. Follow step 6 above.

Sound Meditation

Sound meditation is another simple yet powerful practice, sometimes called *primordial sound meditation*. This may be one of the easier forms of meditation especially for those new the practice, who might have difficulty being in long periods of silence. Sound meditation is a wonderful way to reduce anxiety and stress, expand higher conscious awareness, bring an inner calmness, generate a deep relaxation and impact aligning the five essential components for healing. While research is expanding in the field of sound meditation and therapy, we know that the trillions of atoms and cells making up the tissues of our body are already vibrating and in constant motion. It makes sense then, that the cellular structure of our atoms, already in a state of high-frequency vibration, would be affected and influenced in some way by external sound and vibration.

Sound meditation can be accomplished with percussion sounds, such as drums, gongs or bells, ambient sounds in the form of white noise (static), rustling leaves, ocean waves or rippling streams. Every day outside sounds of any kind can be used for meditation, whether in nature or sounds we might otherwise consider noise, such as, city traffic or jets passing in the sky. Without easy access to nature living in a city and rather than having to join a meditation group with live Tibetan singing bowls, bells and gongs, we have the option of listening to recordings of these instruments.

Sound meditation is best practiced with music having no singing or spoken words that could be a distraction. Listening to instrumental music or focusing on the sound of a bell or singing bowl, without focusing on the sound or making judgements about the music, allows us to transcend our busy, rational mind, bringing us back into the present moment and connection to the Divine.

Sound Meditation:

Step 1.   Start your music or sound.

Step 2.   Sit upright with your hands in your lap, recline or lay comfortably on your back with your arms at your sides and close your eyes. Give yourself a few minutes to get quiet and become aware of your breathing.

Step 3.   You can optionally choose an intention, as an example, focus on healing, relationships, career or any other subject for a working meditation. Another option is simply employing the sound meditation for deep relaxation and rejuvenation. The intention will be your mantra during the meditation.

Step 4.   Shift your awareness, following the stream of sound. Notice if the sound is continuous or if there are silent gaps interrupting the flow. Feel the vibration of the music moving through your body. Notice any sensations in your mind and body that appear as a result of hearing the music or sound. Then refocus your attention, following the sound. Avoid attaching any meaning to the sound.

Step 5. While listening to the sounds, silently repeat your mantra if using this as a working meditation.

Step 6. Over twenty to thirty minutes. Anytime your mind becomes distracted by thoughts or stories in your mind, move your awareness back to your intention or to the sound.

Step 7. Close this meditation by releasing your mantra and gently refocusing your awareness back to the room or space where you sit.

Spend a minute or two being thankful for the serenity of the meditation. Enjoy the elevated sense of peace and well-being.

When you are comfortable, open your eyes.

B. *Progressive Active / Passive Relaxation*

Tight muscles in the body are a common cause of pain and discomfort. This tightness and pain create distractions from our purpose and make difficult aligning the five essential components for healing. Some muscles are chronically tense by the nature of their function. Take the muscles of the spine for instance. Spinal muscles are working throughout the entire day keeping us upright, while controlling bending and twisting. Other times, muscles in the body are often chronically tight as a resulting of emotional tension or occupational postures. In both cases, the brain is constantly sending signals to those muscles maintaining a certain amount of tension. It is quite common for people to have very tight muscles in the neck and upper shoulder (trapezius muscles) region due to anxiety, depression or simply being focused and concentrating on a project. This explains how constant muscle tightness can turn into joint and pain syndromes.

Progressive active / passive relaxation is another mindful practice for reducing muscle tension, lower cortisol levels and relieving stress. This process involves moving your awareness *progressively* through the body, *actively* contracting or tightening muscle groups, holding the tension, then quickly *relaxing* them. During the act of contracting a muscle, our attention is placed on that muscle or group of muscles, acknowledging that they are frequently tight and that we regularly hold tension in that area. In this process, we actively contract muscles making them even tighter than they already are, while focusing on the tightened muscle. By having conscious awareness of the tightened muscles and actively making them over-work, allows us to purposefully and effectively release that tension, thereby letting muscles return to a more normal and relaxed state.

In practicing progressive active / passive relaxation, the idea is to tense each muscle group as intensely as you can without causing pain or injury. During this mindfulness practice, our attention in focused only on the muscle group being contracted and relaxed. We avoid daydreaming or thinking about anything else, always bringing our attention back to the muscle group we are working with. Each muscle contraction is held for approximately five seconds. Avoid producing any pain by intensity or length of contraction. With our mind focused on the actively contracted muscle group, we then make an intentional, sudden release of muscle contraction, visualizing a wave of relaxation and the muscle returning to it's normal, at-rest state. We visualize the muscle in relaxation for several seconds, then repeat a second time or until we feel the muscle group relax, and no more than three times consecutively. Breath normally and avoid holding your breath throughout the exercise. Some like to play music during this exercise.

Progressive active / passive relaxation procedure

- This practice can be accomplished in 15 or 20 minutes.
  Sitting with palms up in your lap or lying down on your back, take your glasses off and place your arms to your sides.
- Take three long, slow Qigong breaths as described in the gratitude meditation, followed by slow Tummo exhales.
- As you begin normal breathing, focus your attention on your feet, toes and ankles.
  Curl your toes and tighten your feet. Hold that tension for approximately three to five seconds.
  Quickly release the tightness and over the next three or four seconds, visualize all the muscles in the ankles, feet and toes, being relaxed and healthy.
  Repeat up to three times or until you feel the muscles relaxed.
- Now move your awareness to the lower legs below the knee and to the ankles. Pulling your toes up toward your head, tighten the muscles around the ankle, muscles of the calf and front of the lower leg. Hold the contraction for three to five seconds.
  Quickly release the tightness and over the following three or four seconds, visualize these muscles of lower leg and ankle released and supple.
  Repeat up to three times or until you feel the muscles relax.
- Moving your focus up to the thighs and knees, contract the muscles in front and back of the thighs (hamstring and quads). Hold for three to five seconds. Quickly release the tightness, while visualizing muscles surrounding the knees and thighs being relaxed over three to four seconds.
  Repeat as above.
- Next, awareness is brought to the muscles of the hips, groin and pelvis. Squeeze the buttock and pelvic floor, holding for three to

five seconds. Quickly release the tightness, focusing on relaxation of these muscles over the following three to four seconds. Repeat.

- Take a long slow deep breath noticing tightness anywhere in your body, releasing all the tension on exhaling.
- Focus your attention now on the lower back and abdomen, tightening the muscles and holding the contraction for three to five seconds.

  Maintaining your focus only on the muscles, quickly release the tension, again visualizing them in their most relaxed state over three to four seconds.

  Repeat.
- Bringing your awareness to the muscles at the front of the chest, take a deep breath, tightening these muscles and holding for three to five seconds. Quickly exhale, releasing all the muscle tension, visualize a wave of relaxation streaming over the muscles of the chest for the next three to four seconds.

  Repeat.
- Move your awareness to your upper back. Take a deep breath while pulling your shoulder blades together, tightening the muscles of the upper back and holding for three to five seconds. Exhale briskly, releasing the tension in these muscles and imaging them being a state of complete rest over three or four seconds.

  Repeat.
- This time, shrug your shoulders up towards your ears, contracting the upper trapezius muscles and holding for three to five seconds.

  Quickly exhale, releasing the muscle tension and visualizing a wave of relaxation pour over the upper trapezius muscles for three or four seconds.

  Repeat.

- Take a deep breath, while exhaling, focus on, and contract the muscles of your shoulders (deltoids and rotator cuff muscles) and upper arms (biceps and triceps), holding that tightness for three to five seconds.
  Quickly exhale, releasing the contracted muscles and focusing on their relaxation for three or four seconds.
  Repeat.
- Take a long, slow deep Qigong breath, hold it for four seconds and slowly exhale, enjoying a wave of relaxation spilling over your body.
- Now bringing your awareness to your forearms, wrists and hands, clench your fists, wrists and tighten your forearms, holding for three to five seconds.
  Quickly let go of the tension, visualizing and feeling a surge of relaxation move through your forearms, hands and wrists over three to four seconds.
  Repeat.
- Breathing in slowly and deep again, exhale, tighten the muscles in your neck and head, holding for three to five seconds.
  On a quick exhale, release all the muscle tension, visualizing your head and neck in a state of complete relaxation over the next three or four seconds.
  Repeat.
- In this last exercise, taking another breath, as you exhale, squeeze your eyes together and scrunch your face in a forced smile, contracting all the muscles of your face. Hold for three to five seconds.
  With a quick release, let all the tightness in your face melt away.
  Repeat.

- Close this practice with three Qigong breaths and Tummo exhales. During this process, notice and appreciate the calm, relaxed state of your entire body and mind.

  Allow yourself five to ten minutes of just being present and in gratitude to the relaxation.

  When you are ready, bring your awareness back to the room and open your eyes.

C. Body-Mind Practices

Qigong, Tai Chi and *yoga* are energy art forms that reduce stress, while at the same time, stimulate the immune system and boost energy centers in the body. As a certified instructor in Qigong Healing Form, a 5,000-year-old energy art ritual, I can tell you that these practices have a profound impact on expanding our healing consciousness. Their practice can be focused specifically on healing while at the same time, promoting energy, clarity and vitality. Teaching any of these mindful practices easily fill entire books and will only be mentioned here. Each of these practices have great value, are available to learn in most cities around the world and with plenty of on-line resources. Not only do these practices stimulate healthful processes in the body and mind, but also create an opportunity for unlocking spiritual connections. Body-mind practices might also include breath empowerment methods and dance.

3. Dream Journaling

"Why does the eye see a thing more clearly in
dreams than the imagination when awake?"

LEONARDO DA VINCI, 15ᵀᴴ/16ᵀᴴ CENTURY PAINTER, SCULPTOR, INVENTOR,

ARCHITECT,

Dreams are not just passive, senseless sleep-time or irrelevant sideshows. Dreams are dynamic, energetic, multidimensional realities during which they present us with symbolic illustrations of our past, present and future. They show us the way we think, feel and behave in our waking life. Dreams are a highly effective ways to address health issues, promote healing and work on any possible waking life issue. Besides Leonardo Da Vinci keeping a dream journal inspiring inventions and designs, dreams have been the acknowledged source of prominent artists, playwrights and musicians from the classical era to rock and roll. Pulitzer Prize authors and politicians have revealed the origin of some ideas and works to have been derived from dreams. Nobel Prize awarded-scientists, have admitted to uncovering their acclaimed new discoveries through knowledge from their dreams. In this section, I am going to show you a practice for healing specific conditions in yourself and others through intentional dream work.

When we dream, our daily subconscious thoughts, judgements and limited thinking are set aside. All waking life distractions are quieted and put on hold. This allows our higher conscious self, a freer and more expansive dream-life experience. Without the obstacles of waking-life thoughts, doors to a multidimensional life perspective opens, permitting an effortless connection to our authentic selves, to our genuine desires and truths. While some people are unable to remember many of their dreams, we know that dreaming occurs every night and that remembering them is a choice. If we are not remembering our dreams, it is probably because we are either too caught up in the wakeful world or would rather not realize their meaning. There is in fact, so much activity, so many experiences and adventures beyond our human comprehension taking place within our dreams, we cannot fully understand them from our earthly perspective. When we do remember a dream, we remember only the tiniest bit of what took place. The part of a dream we remember, is almost always represented symbolically rather than literally, even when there appears to be clear images and literal interpretations. We remember symbols, images or representational stories for a very small portion of an immeasurably vast dream state.

As our authentic thoughts, feelings and intentions present themselves in dreams, it is an ideal tool for understanding our healing consciousness or the healing consciousness of a patient / recipient. In dreams, we can strengthen the energy of our thoughts well beyond our limited, wakeful thinking. It is important to understand that the symbolism of dreams might represent the past, present or future. They may be a narrative for something currently happening in our lives, be premonitions looking forward into the future or a re-experience of an event from the past. In each case, a dream can generate limitations in our lives or inspire us. Working dreams also offer an opportunity for uncovering new, innovative ideas and answers to most any question.

Dreams can be a window into self-imposed obstacles and limitations we have created for ourselves, while at the same time offer solutions for surmounting such blocks and barriers. They can give us insight into any life issues, bringing clarity surrounding business, relationships, career and offer insight into our healing consciousness. A dream can move us in the direction of aligning the five essential components for healing. I call these *working dreams*. American essayist, philosopher and poet, Ralph Waldo Emerson said, "There is one mind common to all man, and having access to this universal mind, you will have access to everything that is and ever was." He believed that through connecting to this universal mind we could connect to anyone from the past and even future. In other words, learn from Plato, Shakespeare or feel what a historical figure felt. Dreams, as in meditation, are avenues to accessing that universal mind Emerson was referring to, connecting with great minds past and present. Through this connection, we can receive tools and guidance towards solutions and accomplishing life goals. Intentional dream work is a powerful instrument for healing, arousing inspiration, discovering innovative ideas and bringing interpersonal clarity in life.

To enhance our skills in dreaming, gain the greatest amount of information and highest benefit, most people will benefit from a practice for remembering and recording their dreams. The following five step, pre-sleep exercise will guide you in developing an intentional dream work practice. Following these steps, will progressively increase the clarity and memory of your dreams. They will also expand the length, enhance images and intensify the experience of dreams.

"I Dream of Painting, Then I Paint My Dream."

VINCENT VAN GOGH, FRENCH IMPRESSIONIST PAINTER

Intentional Dream Work and Dream Recall Exercise

Step 1.   Always keep a *pad of paper and pen* by the bed to record all dream memories as soon as you wake, whether in the middle of the night or first thing in the morning.

Step 2.   Your *Dream Intention*: Once in bed and prior to falling asleep, spend some thoughtful time reflecting a subject for your dream work that night. You might choose a life issue you are struggling with and seeking answers for, guidance taking the next step moving in the direction of a goal or gaining insight related to your career or relationship. When you have a clear subject for your dream, form a statement or question in your mind, concentrating the idea to the least number of clear, focused words that create a powerful affirmation for the work you want to accomplish. The goal is to have this affirmation/intention be the only thought in the deepest recesses of your mind as you fall asleep.

Step 3.   *Dream Declaration*: State your pre-dream affirmation out loud several times and then reaffirm the intention quietly to yourself. This statement or question should be repeated sincerely and powerfully. It might sound something like this: "Tonight, I am going to dream big. It is going to be clear, in color and I am going to remember it in the morning. In this dream I am will *see* (or understand) why... (insert your question or intention)," or "I am going to have insight into the next step in creating... (insert your question or intention)," or "I am going to see what I am supposed to do next with..."

Healing affirmations might include something along the lines of:

"Tonight, my dreams are going to be clear, in color and I'm going to remember them in the morning. I'm going to see the disc and inflammation in my lower back (or my vascular system, liver, lungs, kidneys, whatever the specific health issue is), resorb, the pain go away and the joints return to their normal and healthy state," or "I'm going to have insight for exactly what I need to do to have my... (body area, disease) be healed and fully recovered," or "I'm going to realize the limited thinking and obstacles to healing I have place in my mind that are preventing my recovery."

In other words, affirm to your inner-self that you will gain the clarity you seek on any specific subject in your life.

Step 4. *Solidify Your Declaration*: Be as clear and specific as possible with your intention. Repeat your dream affirmation slowly and clearly over and over until you either fall asleep or *know* beyond words and thoughts that the dream will take place and you will remember it. Repeating the affirmation with sincerity will generate a moment where you know and feel within every cell of your body that without a doubt, you will have this dream and will remember it and record it in your dream journal.

Step 5. *Recording Your Dream*: For many, being consistent in documenting dreams can take significant effort and will power.

Others might wakeup just enough to groggily jot down what they remember then fall back asleep, while still others will pop right up wide eyed, happily recording a dream. The greatest device in developing the habit of dream journaling is in making the effort, immediately taking the step to write, as soon as you have awareness of coming out of a dream. This may not be when you wake in the morning and instead happen during the night. Anytime you wake in the night or on waking in the morning, write whatever you remember from a dream, even if it's just one word. Typically, once you begin to write even that single word, more details unfold. Dreams will become clearer as you write and your ability to remember dreams recalling detail will expand over time. The more you record your dreams, the easier it will be to remember and in greater detail. In a typical night, I commonly experience multiple, large and detailed dreams. Sometimes during the night, it proves easy for me to record dreams and other times it takes great effort to pick-up the dream pad. Either way, I'm always rewarded with the effort.

I cannot stress the importance of writing down any part of a dream you remember, whether waking in the night or first thing in the morning. Each day you make the effort to write down your dreams, the bigger and clearer they become, and the more easily you will remember and record them. You can develop an interesting and healthy habit of dream journaling.

In the process of recording your dreams, there is a natural tendency to figure out what they mean. This will interrupt your memory and clarity of the dream. Instead, keep refocusing your attention on remembering and writing all the details you can remember. Practice letting go of any thoughts of interpretation. Most important is remember what you can and record the details.

Dream Interpretation

My primary intention for including dream work in this book is for its usefulness in expanding healing consciousness and for healing ourselves and others. Learning dream work exercises will likely have made most readers curious about the meaning of their dreams and I want to address some of the basics here. There are a wide range of easily accessible resources for dream interpretation. With some time and effort, it is not difficult to learn these skills.

Here are some basic concepts in understanding dreams. Know that dream interpretations and meaning are unique and specific for every individual. Two people with a similar dream will not have the same interpretation. Dreams are exclusive, filled with individual, intellectual, physical, emotional and spiritual life experience that have accumulated up to the moment of a dream. If you have the references for dream symbology, no one could better interpret a dream than yourself. Remember, dreams are only rarely interpreted literally. In most dreams, people, places, things and environments are symbolic representations of something or someone else associated with your dream intention. When reviewing dream symbolism, you will find that there are many interpretations for each dream symbol. There will almost always be a positive, adverse and neutral explanation for each dream symbol. Avoid being attached to images or circum-stances that are familiar and literal to you, because the interpretation will most likely be completely unrelated. For instance, when there is a person we know in our dream, let's say, a parent, child or friend, and whatever the situation, the significance of their presence in the dream may be to observe a characteristic about them that we see in ourselves. In other words, say, someone we know is bullying us in a dream. The interpretation can be related to seeing ourselves in their anger, maybe wanting to bully or be mad someone else, and most likely not the person in our dream. Another example of how dreams are not interpreted literally, might be when we find ourselves underwater. A dream of being underwater for one person who may feel as if they are drowning, could be a sign of being emotionally overwhelmed or feeling out of control in their life. It could be a sign of suppressed feelings or feeling "underwater," say, financially or in a relationship. Another person having a similar underwater dream, might be comfortably sitting, breathing or swimming under water. This might be a reference to being comfortable as cozy, back in the womb or in control of their emotions and life overall. The point is, while water is the prominent feature of the dream, the way we associate water in our waking life, has little to do with the meaning in our dream.

Once you have awakened and your dream has been recorded, the next step is to look up the meanings for each word, symbol or situation experienced. Read all the possible meanings for each word, symbol or situation in your dream. They will all fit together creating a bigger picture for interpretation. In the process of reading the different meanings, there will come a moment when the correctly associated interpretation "hits home" with you. Along the way of reading positive and adverse meanings, you will have an epiphany of sorts, a physical or emotional reaction to an interpretation that best fits your dream. This will be the case for each word, theme or symbol, putting order to the puzzle of your dream.

Dream work is a powerful place to practice healing and gain inner truths that we may be avoiding. I highly recommend getting into the habit of recording your dreams. If you would like to learn more about my perspective on the power of dreams you might refer to my earlier book "You're Already in Heaven."

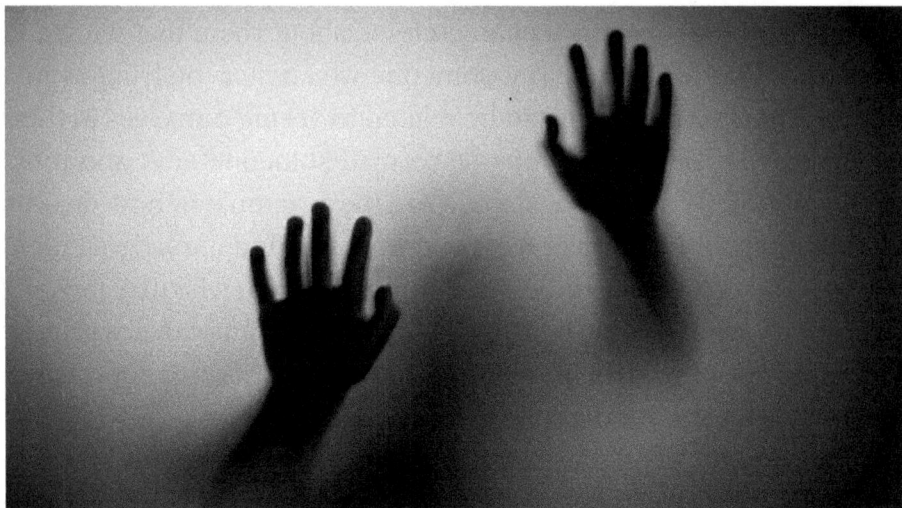

4. Anger, Resentment and Forgiveness Exercise

Anger and resentment cause disease. This is so important, I'm going to repeat it here again. Anger and resentment cause physical, mental and spiritual illness. These emotions also prevent and/or slow healing. We know that negative thoughts and emotions cause stress in the mind and body. They increase circulating levels of cortisol in the blood, disrupt hormonal balance, reduce immune system function, interrupt digestion and reproductive function. These emotions are also known to cause headaches, depression, anxiety, insomnia and heart disease. Anger and resentment are two of the most powerful forms of negative thoughts and emotions. Researchers studying the mind/body connection found stress to shorten life span, permanently alter DNA, many of these practitioners specifically pointing to longtime resentment as a cause of cancer.

Consciously or unconsciously, carrying anger and resentment towards others or for yourself, can cause illness and prevent or delay healing. Examining our underlying, often suppressed, anger and resentment is no easy task, making this one of the most challenging of the writing exercises. At the same time, it can be one of the most compelling and effective practices for removing emotional barriers while promoting alignment of the five essential components for healing. Writing on anger and resentment is an especially powerful practice in reformatting healing consciousness and promoting physical and emotional health.

No one escapes carrying some sort of anger or resentment. Everyone living a normal life, naturally has faced some sort of unpleasant experience and likely more than one, leading to feelings of anger and resentment. They may have been a victim or victimized someone else. There are even situations where someone mistakenly feels victimized, carrying the weight of resentment that may be unjustified and having the same affect. It is likely that most every-one has at some point in their lives, caused someone else discord or pain, even if unintentional. Most people have no conscious inten-tion of doing others harm, though we sometimes inadvertently hurt others or may have been mistakenly perceived by someone else as having caused them some type of wrong doing. This is a typical part of part of living a full life. Ideally, we learn and grow through our mistakes and those of others, doing our best to be conscientious in choosing positive words and behaviors. I point this out not to make judgements or have anyone feeling bad, but rather so that we might find and acknowledge any anger and resentments we carry ourselves. Acknowledgement of our anger and resentment is the first step towards releasing those negative feelings.

Some people might say they have no anger and resentment, or that they have already done all the anger and resentment work nec-essary to be happy. To this, I respond with a question and answer by Mary Morrissey, the renowned business coach and motivational speaker. Mary says, "If you're wondering if you have any anger and resentment work to deal with, ask yourself one question; ask your-self, *am I breathing*? And if the answer is yes, I'm breathing, then the answer is yes, you have anger and resentment work to do." Dealing with anger and resentment is not a one-time affair. We apply anger and resentment work based on our present understanding of the situation and current life perspective. Over time, as we learn and grow, our life perspective changes. When anger or resentment sur-faces related to an old matter, it needs to be addressed once again. Unless we address lingering anger and resentment or whenever it re-emerges, these thoughts and emotions build up, compounding over time and significantly affecting our health.

The key to releasing anger and resentment is *forgiveness*, which is why this exercise is not always easy for some people, especially when they are the result of deeply painful situations. Due to the deeply ingrained nature of anger and resentment, forgiveness is an ongoing process that needs to be revisited when applicable. We forgive based on our current state of awareness in any given moment. Each time we practice forgiveness, by releasing these powerful, destructive thoughts and feelings, extraordinary doors to healing and expanded consciousness can be opened. Forgiveness breaks the cycle of stress in the body and mind that would otherwise trigger cortisol and other harmful biochemicals wreaking havoc on our anatomy and physiology. Practicing forgiveness is calming, reducing stress and anxiety, while promoting harmony, joy and health.

"Forgiveness is the attribute of the strong."

MAHATMA GANDHI

Forgiveness is a mental, emotional and spiritual practice. Even if we never again, saw that person who did us wrong or would avoid a similar situation in the future, we will forever carry anger and resentment in our body and mind without a practice of forgiveness. While we might be holding anger and resentment in our body, being sick or anxious over some stressful life event, the person we blame is not being affected by the way we are feeling. They have probably long forgotten whatever happened and been completely detached from any energy around the event. This leaves only our body and mind to be tormented and ailing. Staying a victim to a past or present event, is giving our power away to others, to someone on the outside, while only causing distress within ourselves. We don't want the wounds of our past to be our identity. In offering authentic forgiveness, we reformat our life perspective in a way that opens the doors of awareness and perception, freeing us to live a life that is unrestricted, one with greater health, purpose and value.

I want to be clear, *forgiveness does not condone poor behavior.* Forgiveness does allow us to release the bindings that keep us attached to a past disparaging situation or person, releasing the associated negative energy that stresses our body and mind, causing illness and delays healing. There is no physical or emotional benefit to carrying anger and resentment towards another person. It keeps *us* locked into the negative feelings and emotions, affecting only our body, minds and spirit. Holding anger and resentment can also be used as an excuse for not taking risks in life. For not being open to relationships, growing a business or developing desired creative endeavors. Forgiveness is the key to releasing anger and resentment.

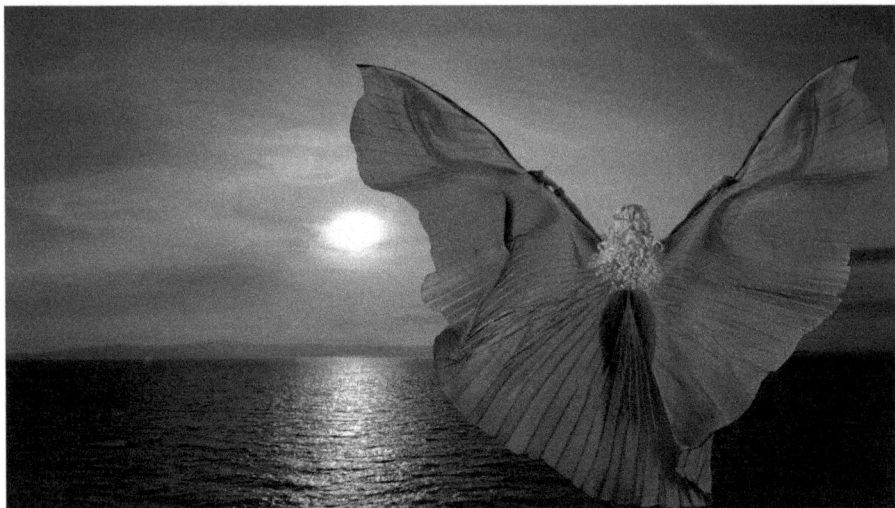

Forgiveness

"Carrying resentment is like a person picking up a hot coal, holding that hot coal and expecting the other person to get burned."

BUDDHA

The first step in forgiving is *acceptance*. Accepting what happened without sticking our heads in the sand and pretending like an event never occurred. Accept the reality of what took place. The second step is to *stop blaming* someone else or blaming yourself for what happened. It happened! Blame will not make anything go away. Blame will only hamper your ability to forgive, while failing to amend a past situation and locking anger and resentment into your mind and heart. No matter what we do, the memory will always be there. The key is removing any active energy surrounding the memory. In other words, allowing the memory to be present, though having no effect on the way we think or feel. Acknowledging and accepting whatever happened, gives us the opportunity to release the negative, unhealthy energy surrounding that person or situation.

In the forgiveness process, we accept what happened, forgive the person or situation, release them and wish them well. This gives us the space to turn our attention toward more creative, healthy and expansive activities in our life, including healing. Additionally, we know that every life event, positive or negative, offer lessons that can be learned about ourselves or human nature. As part of our forgiveness practice, we can find a lesson in every situation, being grateful for expanding our life experience, while further freeing us to move forward and unencumbered in our lives.

"I forgive you for not being the way I wanted you to be. I forgive you and I lovingly set you free."

AUTHOR LOUISE HAY, ON FORGIVENESS

Writing Assignment: The Forgiveness Exercise

The first time you practice this forgiveness exercise, it may be quite time consuming. It is important to write all you can think of on the subject and with as much detail as possible. Each time you practice this forgiveness exercise, it will become easier, quicker and have a deeper and more lasting effect.

Step 1.   Bring to your mind, each person in your life and past events, where you could possibly be carrying anger or resentment. This may be related to family, career, relationships, school, finances, neighbors or friends. Whoever it might be or whatever the situation for holding anger towards them, focus in on the negative *feelings* you carry in your body and mind. Pain, sadness, anxiety, fear, depression, sorrow, anger and resentment are common feelings.

Notice where in your body you hold these feelings. Begin with the ones that take up the greatest amount of energy and attention in your life, the ones that have taken you prisoner in some way, creating emotional blocks and fears. Acknowledge each person and event, writing down, who they are, the situations that took place and all the related feelings you have been holding onto. For each of those people or situations, write the following with meaning, sincerity and know the words to be your truth.

"_____I forgive you and release you for _____
I know I had nothing to do with your behavior and am now free of any obstacles or limitations that kept me bound to that situation. I am free of all anger, resentment, fear or negative energy created by that event.

I take back control of my life and am now free to choose how I will think, feel and act."

Step 2. After finishing this exercise being sure to write this statement for everyone and every situation that comes to mind, the second part of this exercise is forgiving ourselves. Self-forgiveness can have one of the most profound effects in releasing self-imposed obstacles and barriers not only to healing, but in manifesting some of your greatest desires in life.

Most people unconsciously carry some type of anger, resentment or self-judgement about themselves. We humans are so good at compartmentalizing these types of feelings that over time, even though they linger subconsciously, we are rarely cognizant of them. Self-forgiveness might be related to a time we may have hurt someone else or another person having *perceived* that they had been hurt by us, even though it was not our intention. The need to forgive ourselves may come from not having met a life objective or for not completing something we promised ourselves we would do. We may carry anger or resentment towards ourselves around feeling financial or relationship failure. There are countless ways we hold anger or resentment for ourselves.

For this exercise, write the following for as many anger, resentments and self-judgements you might carry for yourself:

"I forgive myself for_____

> I know that I was doing the best I could from where I was, with the resources and knowledge I had at that time.
>
> I know that from this moment forward, I can choose to think and behave in more positive, productive and loving ways toward myself.
>
> I free myself from the past, opening the door to living without limitations.
>
> I am worthy of everything I desire in my life."

Completing these exercises can remove a great amount of weight from your shoulders. You might literally feel lighter, liberated, more courageous and more fully alive. This can be an experience of feeling renewed, living without limitations that produce illness and obstacles to healing, barriers to joy and manifesting your greatest desires. Forgiveness reduces the physical and emotional stresses that create tension in the body. The stresses that raise the levels of cortisol in the blood, disrupt immune system function, hormonal balance, digestion and reproductive health. Forgiveness not only prevents illness but frees our body to heal itself. Further, it brings our mind and body to a place of being susceptible and suggestible to all forms of healing practices. Forgiveness is an important step in aligning the five essential components for healing.

> "Forgiveness is the fragrance the violet sheds
> on the heel that has crushed it."
>
> MARK TWAIN, AMERICAN AUTHOR, HUMORIST, LECTURER

5. Movement and Exercise

Having discussed daily movement and exercise as practice number six, of the six secrets to health, longevity and fitness in the previous chapter, rather than be redundant, I will refer you back to that section of the book. Know that exercise and ideally daily, is important in promoting health, healing and longevity. As with the other tools and exercises in this section, the objective is to expand healing consciousness and support alignment of the five essential components for healing.

"I'm on seafood diet. I see food and I eat it..."

ANON

6. Healthful Eating to Reduce Stress and Disease

As the saying goes, "Eat to live, rather than live to eat." In other words, rather than allowing our emotions, desires or laziness control what we eat, eating to live, means eating when we are hungry, purely to nourish, heal and keep the body and mind healthy. Since nourishing our body and mind are important keys for the efficient function of every cell and organ, and in aligning the five essential components for healing, this section on food and eating will guide you towards healthier living and healing. Healthful eating contributes a great deal to optimizing health, not only through attaining the proper nutrients to run the systems of the body, but also in reducing stress, inflammation, anxiety and elevated cortisol, all contributors to disease and delayed healing. What we ingest will have a direct effect on our ability to align the five essential components for healing. In the last chapter, the first secret to *health, longevity and fitness* is eating close to the farm. In other words, eating, fresh, clean healthy foods, fruits, vegetables and organic meats, while avoiding processed, pre-made foods and sugar. While I'm not going to repeat those guidelines here, you might go back and refresh your understanding of eating close to the farm.

We know that persistent inflammation in the body causes disease. A central contributor to disease related to foods which are very often overlooked, include mild food allergies. The most common effect of a food allergy is both local and general inflammation in the body. This inflammation results from our body considering certain foods to be foreign substances, and in effect, triggering an immune system response. It is not well known that most people, even if very mild, have some form of food allergy. One of the goals in choosing foods for health and healing is to avoid potentially inflammatory foods and instead, opt for those foods that can prevent or reduce inflammation.

Besides having an allergy to a specific food, there are other ingredients associated with processing and the storage of food that can trigger inflammation. These non-food, nutrient absent ingredients, include synthetic chemicals, artificial coloring, non-food flavoring, excessive amounts of sodium, plastics and manu-factured, bio-unavailable preservatives. One of the most prevalent foods causing inflammation and disease is sugar. Beyond sugar and processed foods, it is possible to be allergic to literally any food, even nutrient rich healthy foods. In this section, I am referring to any foods causing inflammation or allergic reactions, and not only speaking about *severe* food allergies. There are the obvious and dangerous allergic food reactions that might cause an anaphylactic reaction, a medical emergency, including symptoms of a skin rash / hives, swelling of the tongue or mouth, nausea, dizziness, vomiting or difficulty breathing. In this case, emergency medical attention is required, along with home care planning and prevention for those who know they have serious food allergies. I'm not talking about these types of serious food allergies. I am referring to instances where even when we are eating mindfully there will be foods that cause mild allergic reactions and inflammation. Symptoms from a mild food allergen might include something as simple as a stuffy nose, a cough, feeling bloated, red or watery eyes, shortness of breath, a mucous film in the mouth or throat, itchy skin, a change in bowel movements as either loose or hard. These are signs that a food or ingredient is causing inflammation in our body. Identifying mild food allergies can be challenging for doctors and patients.

Following is a simple strategy in recognizing food we are sensitive too causing inflammation and potentially disease in our body.

Elimination Diet to Define Food Allergies

We know that serious food allergies can be defined through standard medical testing. But when we're talking about mild food allergies, while there are many medical and alternative tests available, none of them are one hundred percent specific or accurate. These tests often lead to over diagnosis, unnecessary treatment, needless food avoidances, while knowing that food sensitivities change over time. Some children with food allergies eventually grow out of them. People may experience food allergies for the first time as an adult or might have allergic reactions that come and go over time. There are people who become spontaneously sensitized to certain foods, an ingredient in processed foods, a pet, cosmetics or shampoo, triggering their body to be permanently sensitive not only to the initiating ingredient, but also to many other foods or products that were never a problem in the past. The healthiest foods are not exempt from being allergens. Healthy foods that are common, mild allergens for some people, include, tomatoes, strawberries, wheat, eggs and citrus fruit. Mild food allergies create chronic inflammation in the body that will result in anatomical and physiological dysfunction on a cellular level, eventually resulting in illness. Chronic, low-grade inflammation in the body can be a killer.

As most people fail to realize mild food allergies that generate significant adverse health effects, one way to ascertain a simple food allergy would be to undertake an *elimination diet*. In an elimination diet, all possible allergic foods are avoided over a four-week period. Eliminate from the diet any food you believe causes a mild allergic reaction in your body. Common foods to avoid during the four-week elimination period might include:

All processed foods including but not limited to, precooked foods/meals, baked goods, dressings and sauces.

Processed meats	Sugar	Dairy	Chocolate
Wheat	Eggs	Tomato	Corn
Fried Foods	Beer / Wine	Preservatives / Additives	

Following the four-week elimination period for these foods, to ascertain a food allergy, add one food at a time back into your diet over a three-day period. Choose a food you miss the most and eat larger than typical quantities over a three-day period. While reintroducing these foods back into your diet one at a time, practice mindful eating, exercising keen body awareness, noticing even the simplest signs or symptom allergic reactions as described above. Any mild allergic reactions to the re-introduced foods, will tell you that you have a sensitivity to that food, meaning it is likely producing inflammation in your body. Through mindful eating, some people can identify those mild allergic reactions without using an elimination diet. If we are listening, our body knows which foods to eat and those to avoid. I know that dairy products, wine and beer having been fermented in yeast or hops, and sugar are mild allergens causing a reaction in my body.

It is important to understand that this elimination diet is a tool for determining only *mild food allergies* that over time, can develop and promote, chronic dis-ease causing inflammation in the body. In other words, its function is to identify foods that we commonly eat, even consider healthy, though have the ability in some people to generate chronic inflammation leading to disease. On the other hand, a small percentage of the population have *serious food allergies* that can be life threatening and require proper medical care.

Peanut allergies for example, can be life threatening and a great concern for parents with children, but statistics show that they occur in only 0.4-0.6% percent of the population. Less than one percent. Gluten sensitivity which seems to have gained unwarranted attention, has been identified in only four percent of the population. The bottom line is, to know that acute care and lifetime medical attention is essential for the diagnosis and prevention of serious food allergies, while mild food allergies are quite common. Most medical data agree on a list of eight or ten foods being the most frequently associated with serious food allergies, triggering serious or life-threatening allergic reactions. Those foods include but are not limited to:

| Milk | Wheat | Shellfish Fish | Peanuts |

Tree Nuts (walnuts, pine nuts, almond, Brazil nuts, pecans)

| Soy | Eggs |

Mild food allergens are much more common and extend beyond the typical serious food allergy lists. These milder food allergens, the ones we can eat with very tolerable and sometimes imperceptible amounts of discomfort, are the ones that initiate chronic inflammation in the body. Chronic inflammation over time, causes disease and dysfunction within the body. Milk and dairy products are probably the most common mild food allergens. It is not uncommon though, to be mildly allergic to milk and certain cheeses, while not being sensitive to yogurt or some hard cheeses, where the casein (mild protein) and lactose (milk sugar) has been broken down. Similarly, while some people might be allergic to raw eggs and more commonly the protein in the egg whites, may at the same time, not be allergic to cooked eggs. Most children grow out of allergies to eggs. The bottom line is in understanding that we can learn which foods are unique allergens for ourselves, causing chronic inflammation in our body and eventually disease. This allows us to avoid those foods and boost our ability to heal and be healthy.

For your reference, following are two lists, one of foods that commonly cause inflammation in the body and a list of foods that reduce inflammation. You will notice that there are a few foods on both the inflammatory / allergen food list, also present on the anti-inflammatory list. That is because as previously noted, some people have mild allergies to foods we typically consider healthy and can be identified through the elimination diet or medical testing. These lists are designed to help you create a healthy, anti-inflammatory eating habit. For optimal health, which is part of the knowledge and understanding in aligning the five essential components for healing, it is important for you identify foods that are particularly inflammatory to your unique anatomy and physiology, so that you can avoid them as best as possible.

The most common "mild" food allergens (serious to some) causing acute or chronic inflammation in the body:

Sugar

Dairy Products (yogurt and hard cheeses may be an exception for some people)

Beer and Wine (allergens: hops, yeast and tannins)

All Artificial Sweeteners and Natural Processed Sweeteners

Chocolate

Shellfish

Tree Nuts

Soybeans

Peanuts

Foods considered healthy that some people have mild allergies to:

Tomatoes	Wheat / Gluten	Barley	Strawberries
Citrus	Eggs	Eggplant	
Bananas	Avocado	Kiwi Fruit	Peach
Red Meat	Corn	Mango	

Flour: Refined / Processed Grains

With or without a mild food allergy, a general rule in reducing inflammation in the body, would be to avoid all processed sugar, processed foods and eating organic to avoid pesticides when possible.

Barring signs of allergies, the following foods can reduce inflammation in the body, lower cortisol levels in the blood and reduce stress:

Almonds	Avocado	Beets	Blueberries	Broccoli
Cabbage	Cal-Mag	Carrots	Cashews	Celery
Chard	Cherries	Chia Seeds	Chocolate Dark (1.4 oz/day)	
Cinnamon	Coconut Oil	Coffee	Eggs	Flax Seeds
Garbanzo Beans	Ginger	Green Leafy Vegetables		
Whole Grains (not whole grain flour)			Green tea	Kale
Lemon	Lemon Balm	Lentil Beans	Nuts	Nutmeg
Oatmeal	Omega 3 Fatty Acids		Oranges	Papaya
Peppermint	Peppermint Tea		Pineapple	Pistachio Nuts
Pumpkin Seeds	Raisins	Raspberries	Salmon/Tuna/Sardines	
Spinach	Sprouted Seeds		Sunflower Seeds	
Sweet Potatoes	Winter Squash		Swiss Chard	
Turkey Breast	Turmeric	Valerian Root		
Vitamin C	Walnuts	Yogurt (sugar free)	Lysine & Arginine	

Whenever possible choose organic fruits and vegetables as they readily absorb pesticides, not only in their skins, but within the substance of the food. Especially vulnerable, with potentially more than thirty pesticides present in a crop, are apples, strawberries, all berries, cherries, cucumbers, grapes, lettuce, nectarines, peaches, peanuts, pears, potatoes, tomatoes, spinach and sweet bell peppers. Avoiding food allergens will contribute significantly to general health, healing of injuries, illness and aligning the five essential components for healing.

"Music has healing power. It has the ability to take people out of themselves."

ELTON JOHN, SINGER, PIANIST, COMPOSER

7. Sound Therapy

In the last chapter I described a meditation practice using sound. Sound therapy differs from sound meditation in that sound is being applied passively to our mind and body, in order to move our anatomy and physiology in healing directions. Sound therapy actively employs music or tones for healing purposes, while a sound meditation is a tool for becoming centered and calm. This will better explain, the way Sound Therapy functions as another avenue for reducing stress and cortisol, making it an additional instrument for aligning the five essential components for healing. Sound and vibration effect and move the already vibrating cells of the body. Think about the way music alters our thoughts and feelings. A song might have us feeling excited, happy, elated or dreamy. Music might move us to feel anxious, distressed, sad, sorrowful or fearful. The music and sound effects for movies, are designed to have us think and feel in a very specific manner that occurs through changing our physical vibration on a cellular level.

In medicine, music therapy termed *music intervention,* is now considered a viable treatment. Music intervention is being used for pre-operative anxiety, which has been associated with negative physical manifestations, such as, slow wound healing, increased chance for infection, complications under anesthesia and delayed recovery. Sound therapy includes, passive listening to pleasant music, meditating on a sound or song, singing or playing an instrument. The listening during sound therapy takes place not only in the mind, but also by every cell in the body. Music therapy can be accomplished through sounds of nature, such as, the ocean against the shoreline, a water fountain, waterfall or rustling of leaves in a breeze. Part of the effects of music therapy include what is called *the vibroacoustic effect.* The theory is that the frequency of sound waves alters the vibration of the atoms in our cells. This activation of our cells by sound, renders them susceptible to modifications in treatment by both medicine and healing methods. At minimum, music therapy can reduce anxiety, lower blood pressure and elevated cortisol, slow heart rate and reduce muscle tension. Sound can elevate one's mood, reduce pain and discomfort. Music Therapy is also said to reduce the intensity of dementia, aid in speech therapy, improve the quality of life and create a general sense of well-being. Enjoying the sounds of nature, pleasant, positive or joyful music, will contribute to expanding healing consciousness and aligning the five essential components for healing.

8. Journaling

Journaling is a powerful method for gaining clarity, removing limited thinking, expanding healing consciousness and aligning the five essential components for healing. In the beginning of this chapter, I presented writing exercises specifically geared towards removing blocks and barriers to healing, and in releasing negative thinking around present illnesses. Here, I present journaling exercises as an effective method for reducing stress, gaining focused perspective on life issues, reducing cortisol and calming the mind and body. These are all attributes of expanding healing consciousness and aligning the five essential components for healing.

For centuries, scientists, politicians and business leaders have been journaling not only for documentary purposes, but also as a problem-solving tool or aiding in the evolution of new ideas. Journaling can propagate a positive influence on physical and mental health, reducing inflammation, boosting the immune system and elevating our mood. In putting our thoughts and feelings to paper, not only can we quickly gain clarity on life issues, but, reduce the emotional and physical effects of traumatic experiences. Journaling can be structured by focusing on definitive subjects, questions, guidance toward intentions or simply *stream of consciousness* writing. When we write organically, without intention, whatever comes to mind and on any subject, we are practicing stream of consciousness writing.

For more journaling ideas, rather than be redundant, look back to the sections on writing related to illness, forgiveness and especially gratitude. The following is an example of writing for clarity on life issues, expanding healing consciousness or growing new ideas. This type of journaling is a freeing, unreserved practice that can be quite revelatory, further opening the door to aligning the essential components for healing.

Stream of Consciousness Writing

Writing in this manner will reveal and develop new concepts, bringing fresh perspectives we may have over looked or avoided, and brings clarity to old or ongoing life issues. This type of journaling can also remove redundant thoughts, useless toiling of hardships and ordeals, putting them onto paper and out of your head. In stream of consciousness writing, you can choose an initial thought / subject (a new idea, relationships, career, school, family) or freely begin writing with whatever is most prevalent, on your mind. There is an unobstructed truth that arises out of this type of writing that may bring surprises to the paper. To utilize stream of consciousness writing, begin with a single word, a question or an idea. Without trying, without judgement of what you might pen and with no editing, simply write everything that comes to mind. This type of writing does not have to make sense, does not have to be orderly or harmonious, you just write. While there is no time limit on how long you might journal, spend at least fifteen to twenty minutes writing.

Most often, thoughts expand, new ideas form, old ideas transmute, and order ensues, generating inner excitement, inspiration and valuable results. If new discoveries evolve through your writing, further develop them through outlines and greater detail. You may be inspired to action in resolving life challenges, taking steps on a current venture or launching a new project. By the end of your journaling, you will be feeling lighter, brighter, more focused and have an elevated sense of well-being. Stream of consciousness writing is an enjoyable, worthwhile, consciousness expanding and healing experience.

Gratitude Journaling

This last journaling exercise on *gratitude* is designed to bring healing to every aspect of your mind and body while lifting your spirits. Like the gratitude meditation, this is an exercise bringing you to the realization that you have everything you will ever need to be happy and that joy is conscious choice in any given moment. Gratitude journaling breaks patterns of negative thinking about difficulties in life. Rather than toiling over life's challenging issues, you can journal yourself to joy and healing.

1. Make a list of *at least* twenty basic life comforts you are grateful for, such as, having a roof over your head, food on the table, change in your pocket, a bed to sleep in or additional creature comforts you might be taking for granted.

2. Make a list of at least five life situations you are grateful for, maybe, having family, a job, friends, etc.

3. Write about at least three of the most important people in your life and why you are grateful for them.

4. Make a list of anything that makes you happy in your life.

9. Stress and Healing Reduction Through Intimacy

Intimacy: *A close, familiar and affectionate or loving relationship with another person or group.*

Human connection, touch and companionship can be significant contributors to reducing stress, anxiety and lowering cortisol levels. In his book, *"The Seven Principles for Making Marriage Work,"* John M. Gottman, PhD, notes that happily married couples are more health conscious and live longer than those who are not. He also describes his latest research findings pointing to a good marriage giving the immune system an extra boost. Connection, love, intimacy, compassion and empathy, all support the healing process. Intimacy can be intellectual as with friends, colleagues and relationships, it might be emotional as with a parent, child relationship and with partners. Intimacy can also be spiritual or sexual, as with an intimate relationship. Under fitting circumstances, human touch triggers calming and stress reduction. A parent and child or couple holding hands creates an intimate calming, loving and healing bond. Cuddling a pet can generate calm and healing. In partnerships / relationships, kissing, touching, being vulnerable and making love, not only reduce stress and promote healing, but deepens the union between couples. Laughing and dancing creates human connection and being in service to others can also create an intimate connection that reduces stress and supports healing in the body.

This completes the practices and exercises for expanding healing consciousness and aligning the five essential components for healing. Each of these practices alone, contribute to altering the way you understand illness and beliefs regarding how healing is supposed to take place. Many of the mindful tools together, can empower you towards further developing the skills in healing yourself and others, while generating more joy and harmony in your life.

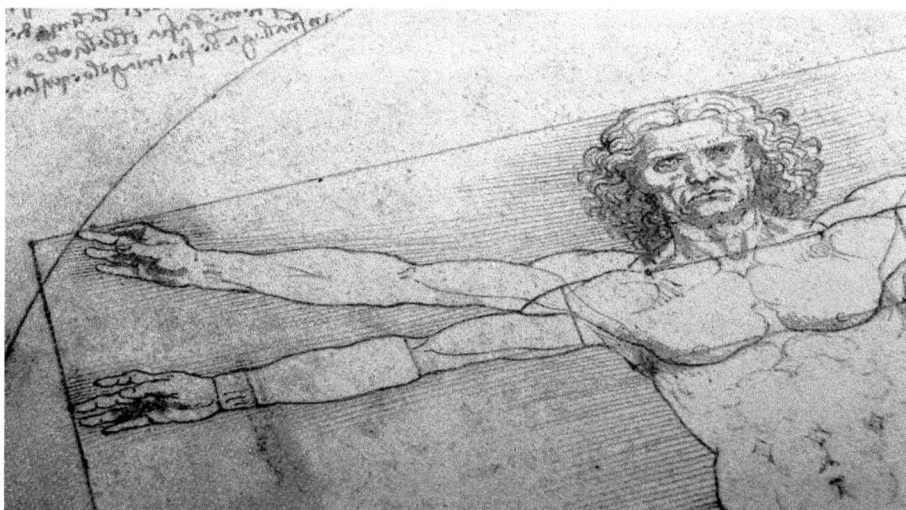

CHAPTER SEVEN

A New Paradigm In Healing

Having arrived at the final chapter, know that consciously, anatomically and physiologically, you are not the same person you were when you began reading this book. Your genetic coding, the DNA in your chromosomes, have been permanently reformatted with expansive, positive perspectives and new understandings of illness and the countless possibilities for healing to take place. By guiding you through "*The Five Secrets for Healing Yourself and Others*," your healing consciousness has been permanently modified, paving the way for intentionally and purposefully achieving the state of *knowing*, without a doubt, that you will heal. You have had and now carry with you, the opportunity for releasing and reformatting many of the limiting thoughts and emotions preventing or delaying healing. Your capacity to more easily heal yourself and others has been enduringly broadened and enhanced. These tools you have received tools, can bring you greater health, longevity, fitness and joy.

All too often when faced with illness, people become over-whelmed, obsessed or emotionally paralyzed. They are consumed with trying to figure out what they *believe* is the real problem, beyond even what doctors have told them. This can take them down an almost endless path of worry, anxiety and fear to the point of man-ufacturing new, inaccurate thoughts and feelings regarding illness or even new dis-ease. This type of health obsession is fueled by an irresistible submersion into the volumes of confusing information, mis-representation, bias and even unscrupulous on-line informa-tion by self-professed experts. Do not let your health be hacked by the internet. We also want to avoid any obsessive and compulsive thoughts and behaviors around health, even positive thoughts, such as, *trying* to be better or healthier. Being consumed and controlled by illness in both positive or negative ways, can disrupt our lives, interfere with daily activities, work, family and relationships, reduc-ing our productivity and the ability to meet our daily needs.

Our intentions would serve us better by being focused on tran-scending the myopic distress of obsessing on disease. With this new knowledge you have gained on healing, rather than being a slave to insurance companies, doctors and illness, the time has come to take control of your own health and healing. Fortunately, it is somewhat easier in these times to be an active participant in our healthcare. While by small steps, there is a positive global shift in health management, along with the rapid growth and recognition of alternative, natural healthcare and healing methods. Many allopathic physicians have finally taken steps towards a more holistic approach to patients. Doctors are being more mindful and creative in their diagnostic and therapeutic approaches, focusing on the unique individuality of each patient. My hope is that physicians are becoming more accessible, listening closely, having more patience in answering questions and making referrals for treatments that might be out of their area of expertise, including alternative therapies. As this is a slow transformation for physicians, most doctors will still not initiate these actions on their own. It is our responsibility and a gift to ourselves that we make deliberate efforts in being active participants in our healthcare. Think of a visit with your doctor as an obligation to yourself, for asking questions, fully understanding what they are telling you regarding your condition, the reason for a prescribed treatment and what other therapy options are available.

No one should feel intimidated in asking all the questions they need answered by their physicians. The better the understanding of your condition and treatment, the greater the trust in the practitioner and the more likely the five essential components for healing will be aligned. It is time to be a proactive partner with your doctor in making the best choices for your healthcare. Broadening your healing consciousness to the greater potentials and opportunities in a cure, beyond the limitations you used to believe were the only possibilities, will bring you to that place of knowing you will heal without a doubt. Always do everything you possibly can when addressing any health condition. In addition to your doctor's care, this may include, alternative therapies not readily suggested by your physician due limitations of their knowledge in these other avenues for treatment. You never know unless you ask.

Remember that when it comes to ill-health and healing, we are always thinking and acting from our current level of understanding, awareness and truth. When facing ill health, expanding our knowledge, understanding, belief, faith and non-attachment to outcome is an ongoing evolution. A revolution in releasing stuck and rigid, ineffective ways of thinking and being. If this is your first time reading my book or one like it, let this be a call to action in your process of becoming more conscious, better informed, healthier and more skilled at healing. One of the greatest gifts we have is our ability to increasingly raise our consciousness. You now have this opportunity to further develop and broaden your healing consciousness. This is a chance for you to be an active participant, in reformatting the way you have been automatically thinking about illness and health. Expansion of your healing consciousness elevates your overall state of well-being, generating greater vitality and energy to your life adventure. Following mindful practices and working towards aligning the five secrets for healing, you will possess and express greater joy for yourself and those around you.

Recent studies of centenarians, those living longer than 100 years, showed several commonalities. They found that these individuals were lifelong learners. They were active, being in service (volunteering) and participating in creative activities. All of them considered connections with family and/or friends important. The majority had outgoing cheerful life attitudes, and none exhibited hostile or neurotic personalities. They all tended to avoid conflicts. These centenarians exercised and enjoyed art, culture and sex. While their diets varied depending on region, they enjoyed eating and drinking in moderation, primarily consuming fresh, unprocessed foods. These centenarians are all innately aligned with mindful, conscientious practices.

The intention of this book has been to reveal the foundation for all healing, inspiring you in your ability as an active participant and healer of yourself and others. In that process, I described how learned limitations and bias regarding the way we *believe* healing takes place, affects our health and ability to heal. I offered tools in reformatting those limited thoughts and beliefs, replacing that information with more expansive understandings for the nature of illness and health. In other words, we jump-started expansion of your healing consciousness. Continue cultivating acceptance that healing can take place in ways you never imagined. For some readers, this book may have provided order to thoughts and feelings they knew subconsciously, but had been unable to organize in meaningful, applicable procedures and practices. My goal is to enhance your already innate ability to heal yourself and others, whether from the simplest cut on a finger to what you might have thought was a most frightful illness.

This new paradigm in expanded healing consciousness is designed to be part of your everyday, automatic thought process and behavior, in relation to the way you perceive illness and how you *know* healing can unfold. The book concludes with practical practices and exercises designed to be healing consciousness altering, contributing to the alignment of the five essential components for healing and leading to new possibilities in healing any condition. The regular practice of meditation, dream work, journaling, healthful eating, movement and exercise, will significantly compound your ability to take charge of your healing process, be part of healing others and living with greater health and well-being. Recognize the benefit in revisiting the writing exercises, especially journaling around illness, anger and resentment, practices that will continue to release subconscious limitations and obstacles while improving your healing skills and broaden your healing consciousness.

Remember that healing from any dis-ease or being in optimal health always comes back to the way we are thinking. As I teach in my healing retreats and as one of the principal foundations in my practice of BioCognitive Healing, "Thoughts change biochemistry." And you now know that every one of those 80,000 thoughts we have each day, triggers chemical reactions in the body. If these thoughts are negative, narrow and jammed with limitations, negative, unhealthy changes will take place in the body, such as, chronic inflammation and persistently elevated levels of cortisol. On the other hand, if our thoughts are positive, expansive and without barriers, their physical and energetic nature will stimulate positive, healthy and healing effects on the body, triggering the immune system, specific glands, tissues and organs, promoting healing. From our healing consciousness comes the commanding, energetic nature of our thoughts required for healing, that align the five essential components and bring us to that place of *knowingness*, where without any doubt, we are going to heal. This is the moment when the administrative energy of our thoughts, alters our biochemistry, generating the greatest effects of all healing on the body.

I hope this book inspires you to continue opening your mind, expanding your healing consciousness and heart to the greater possibilities in healing. That you will choose to take a more proactive approach to your healthcare and greater action in your own healing through the way you think, feel and move towards aligning the five essential components. It should now be clear that the energy of your thoughts, feelings and emotions alter the chemistry in your body, creating either imbalance and potentially leading to illness or stimulating your body's natural ability to heal itself.

By continuing to follow guidelines and practices in this book, there will be an evolution in your ability to healing yourself and others. No longer will you be resigned to passivity in your own healing or be enslaved by backwards models of healthcare. Understanding *"The Five Secrets for Healing Yourself and Others,"* represents a shift in the healing paradigm. It is a leap forward in our ability to consciously, intentionally and purposefully, heal ourselves and others. From this time forward, be part of expanding the healing consciousness not only of yourself, but for your family, friends and the world around you. Exercise compassion, elevating and guiding others towards their greater possibilities in healing and contributing to health and joy in the world.

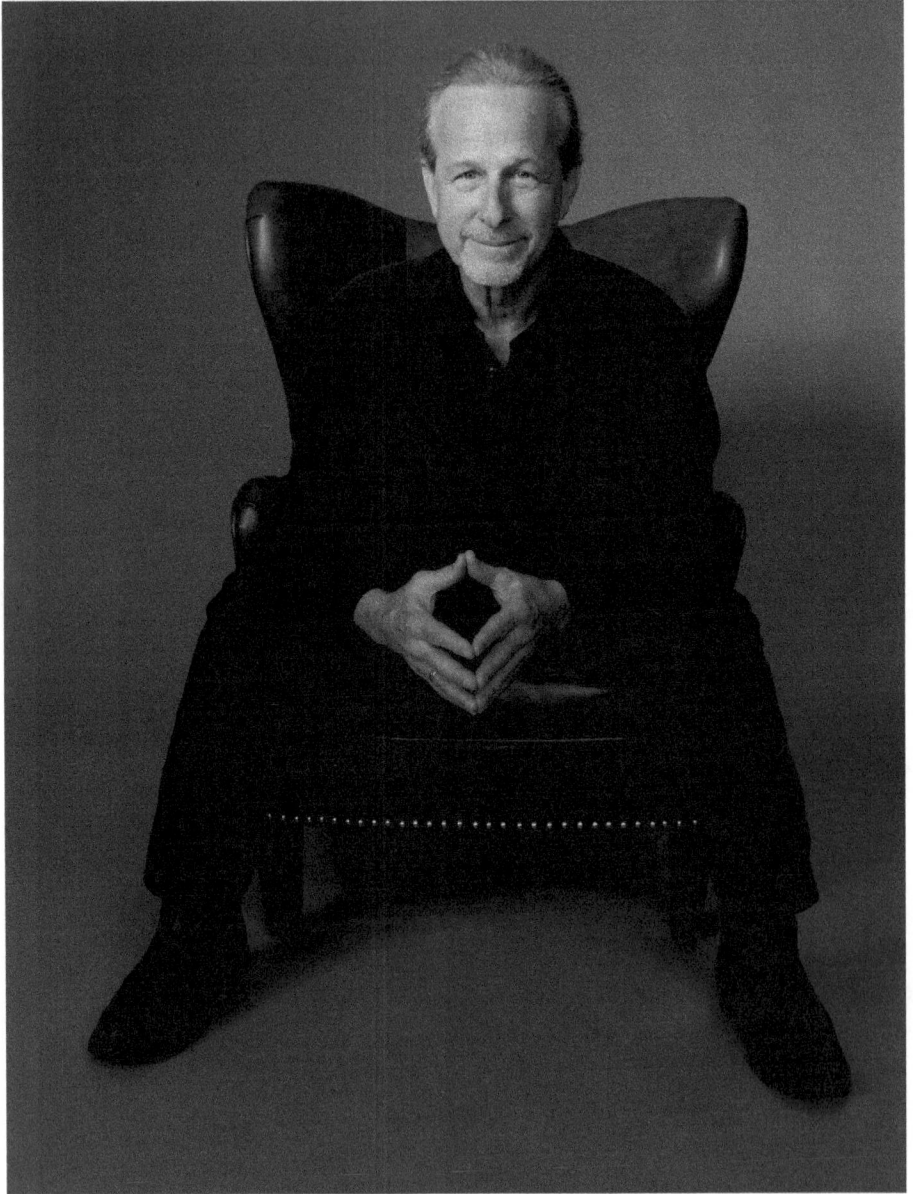

About the Author

D r. Futoran practiced Chiropractic Orthopedics in Studio City, California for more than 30 years, served as president of the American College of Chiropractic Orthopedists and as an examining commissioner on State, National and specialty orthopedic boards. He has lectured internationally on numerous clinical subjects, published professional papers and was instrumental in developing ultrasound imaging for neuromusculoskeletal diagnosis. With more than forty years of experience in the healing arts, he now leads Longevity, Mindfulness and Healing retreats internationally. Dr. Futoran is a practicing Health and Mindset Coach. He is additionally certified in Hypnotherapy as a Qigong instructor and has developed and teaches the Bio-Cognitive Healing Method.

www.ingramcontent.com/pod-product-compliance
Lightning Source LLC
Chambersburg PA
CBHW070927030426
42336CB00014BA/2562